EPSOM SALT

150 Extraordinary Natural Remedies,
Uses, and Benefits for Your Health,
Body, Beauty, & Home

Contents

WHAT IS EPSOM SALT?

Epsom Salt was discovered hundreds of years ago (in 1618) in a water spring in Epsom, a village in Surrey (England) after a farmer discovered that although his cows were unhappy with the bitter taste of spring water which they drunk, they were healed of their rashes and scratches. The good news about this miracle product soon spread and it began to be prepared by boiling down spring water, which contained porous chalk material from North Downs (UK) combined with non-porous clay silt from London. This combination resulted in the creation of a crystal like mineral containing magnesium and sulfur which is today referred to as the Epsom Salt.

Epsom salt is also known as magnesium sulfate and is considered as a pure, naturally occurring mineral compound with some amazing healing and beautifying properties.

Since the mineral is quick to absorb water and bacteria, it was commonly used by doctors all over the world to sanitize medical tools and instruments.

Epsom Salt is also included in the World Health Organization's Model List of Essential Medicines (owing to its numerous uses).

The common society still uses it as a bath salt, and it is a favorite with athletes aspiring to relieve themselves from muscle aches and pains.

As you read through the book, you will get to understand the various uses of Epsom Salt which make it much more than just an added luxury in your bath salt.

Besides its ability to heal the body from many physical ailments and health conditions, Epsom Salt also boasts of several household, beautifying, detoxifying, and gardening related benefits.

THINGS TO REMEMBER BEFORE GETTING STARTED

Some people may get a reaction from magnesium – it may lead to a stomach upset or other complications if consumed in large, unsafe amounts. Always consult a doctor if you suspect that you are unwell.

Consult with a qualified medical practitioner and/or doctor before using Epsom Salt and the recipes provided in this book. In case you suffer from any medical condition, allergies, or are pregnant. Readers who fail to consult with appropriate health authorities assume and are responsible for the risk of any injuries. The respective authors and publisher are not liable.

This book is meant for informational purposes only. It is NOT intended to be used as a medical source. This book is NOT meant to be a substitute for medical advice. This book is NOT meant to be taken over any advice provided by your doctor or medical professional. This health book is NOT intended to be used for diagnosing or treating a problem or disease. The natural health information have NOT been evaluated by any statutory or professional body and are not intended to diagnose, treat, cure, or prevent any disease.

Never go overboard with Epsom Salt and use only the recommended dose as and when needed.

Never let your pets consume Epsom Salt.

Always ensure that the type of Epsom Salt you are using contains magnesium sulfate as its main ingredient.

Never use Epsom Salt on children below six years of age.

Before you get started with Epsom Salt, use wisely and with caution, especially if you are using it for healthcare.

If you are a diabetic or suffer from dry, cracked or fragile skin, use gentle foot soaks instead of a full body soak.

If you are using all the precautions mentioned above, nothing can be as miraculous as Epsom Salt. This book covers 150 amazing uses of Epsom Salt. These uses have been divided into various categories but have been numbered by serial order.

Feel free to use this miraculous salt as a part of your daily, bath, beauty, health, DIY recipes, cleaning or gardening routine.

Please note that the recipes in this book are

Ready to get started?

Let's go!

USING EPSOM SALT FOR HEALTH

Epsom Salt can be great for your overall health. Incorporating it into your daily, weekly or fortnightly health routine is not only amazingly easy and convenient but also a safe, natural and affordable way to relieve common ailments and stimulate your body's natural immunity.

Here are some awesome Epsom Salt recipes:

USE 1: FLU RELIEF VIA EPSOM SALT

Do you want to reap the immune strengthening benefits of Epsom Salt? All you need to do is to soak yourself in this relaxing, effective and simple flu-fighting remedy.

Simply add 2 cups of Epsom Salt, 1 cup Baking soda, 5 drops of Eucalyptus essential oil, 7 drops of Tea tree essential oil, 4 drops of ginger essential oil in a tub full of warm water. Soak for at least 30 minutes.

USE 2: ANTI FLU BATH

Heard about the miraculous benefits of green tea? It is loaded with immunity strengthening anti-oxidants that enable your cells to fight off the germs which are making you sick.

List of ingredients:

- 1 cup Green tea (steeped for five minutes)
- 1 cup Epsom Salt
- 1 tbsp. Garlic powder
- 10 drops Peppermint essential oil
- 5 drops Lavender essential oil
- A tub full of Warm water

Directions:

Add all the ingredients in the tub and soak body in bath for at least 20 minutes.

USE 3: LEMON AND EPSOM SALT BATH FOR FIGHTING COMMON COLD AND FLU

Ginger is a natural decongestant and lemon give this bath an amazing freshness.

List of ingredients:

- Juice of 1 Lemon
- 1 cup Epsom Salt
- 2 inch Ginger root (powdered or very thinly sliced)
- 10 drops Tea tree essential oil
- A tub full of Warm water

Directions:

Add all the ingredients in the tub and soak body in bath for at least 20 minutes.

USE 4: SOOTHING BATH SOAK FOR PAINS AND ACHES

This soak is extremely effective in case you are experiencing tired or fatigued muscles or even pain in joints. The Lavender essential oil used in the soak helps you beat all stress and relax.

List of ingredients:

- 1 cup Epsom Salt
- 10 drops Lavender essential oil
- A tub full of Warm water

Directions:

Add all the ingredients in the tub and soak body in bath for at least 20 minutes.

USE 5: ANTI INFLAMMATORY SOAK

The combination of Chamomile and magnesium sulfate make this bath soak extremely relaxing and anti-inflammatory too.

List of ingredients:

- 1 cup Epsom Salt
- 10 drops Chamomile essential oil
- 10 drops Sweet Marjoram essential oil
- 1 tsp. Cinnamon powder
- A tub full of Warm water

Directions:

Add all the ingredients in the tub and soak body in bath for at least 20 minutes.

USE 6: PMS SOOTHING SOAK

Chamomile essential oil used in combination with Epsom Salt is great to soothe symptoms of PMS.

List of ingredients:

- 1 cup Epsom Salt
- 15 drops Chamomile essential oil
- A tub full of Warm water

Directions:

Add all the ingredients in the tub and soak body in bath for at least 20 minutes. Do not rinse off – just towel dry and wrap yourself in a warm blanket for at least thirty minutes after the soak.

USE 7: PAIN RELIEVING BATH SOAK

Epsom Salt has been since time immemorial to relieve aches and pains. It helps in soothing stiff muscles and becomes even more impactful when used in combination with Eucalyptus, Peppermint and Clary Sage essential oils.

List of ingredients:

- 1 cup Epsom Salt
- 10 drops Eucalyptus essential oil
- 5 drops Clary Sage essential oil
- 5 drops Peppermint essential oil
- A tub full of Warm water

Directions:

Add all the ingredients in the tub and soak body in bath for at least 20 minutes.

USE 8: ANTI SPSMODIC BATH SOAK

This recipe uses Thyme and Rosemary essential oils which elevate the anti-spasmodic properties of Epsom Salt.

List of ingredients:

- 1 cup Epsom Salt
- 10 drops Thyme essential oil
- 10 drops Rosemary essential oil

- 1 tsp. Cumin powder
- A tub full of Warm water

Directions:

Add all the ingredients in the tub and soak body in bath for at least 20 minutes to experience instantaneous relief from muscle spasms, back ache and stomach ache.

USE 10: ANTI ARTHRITIC BATH SOAK

This recipe uses Ginger essential oil which not only eases back pain and enhances mobility but also treats rheumatic and arthritic pains, muscle spasms and sprains.

List of ingredients:

- 1 cup Epsom Salt
- 10 drops Ginger essential oil
- 5 drops Lavender essential oil

- 1 tsp. Cinnamon powder
- A tub full of Warm water

Directions:

Add all the ingredients in the tub and soak body in bath for at least 20 minutes. Repeat this every day for at least a fortnight to experience amazing arthritic relief.

USE 11: ARTHRITIC RELIEF VIA EPSOM SALT

Simply soaking your body in three cups of Epsom Salt dissolved in a tub full of warm water can help you get rid of a debilitating condition called arthritis.

This remedy is a lot cheaper than many commercially available products. You can even use it selectively. Want to help the pain in your hands? Soak in a bowl of Epsom salt infused warm water.

Use some lemon essential oil to add a dash of instant energy.

USE 12: EPSOM SALT BLOOD SUGAR CONTROLLER

Research proves that low levels of magnesium in the body have a major role to play in diabetes and insulin resistance. An occasional dose of minerals via the Epsom Salt helps in regulating the blood sugar level and improving insulin resistance. All you need to do is drink a glassful of Epsom salt infused filtered water. Add a tablespoon of Epsom Salt to one glass filtered water. Drink slowly and then drink a glass of pure, unadulterated filtered water to get rid of the after taste. Use this remedy only after consulting your medical practitioner.

USE 13: INSULIN REGULATOR

In order to help with insulin resistance, you may occasionally add a tablespoon of Epsom Salt to a cup of Peppermint tea. Drink this slowly to soothe yourself and experience long term blood sugar regulation.

Once again, do not use it without the guidance of a registered medical practitioner.

USE 14: BATH TO SOOTHE NERVE PAIN AND CRAMPS

The main thing that leads to decreased nerve and muscle function is fluid retention. This can be dramatically improved through the magnesium sulfate content in Epsom salt. Soak yourself in a tub full of warm water that has 2 cups Epsom Salt, 10 drops Rosemary essential oil and 5 drops Tea tree essential oil added to it.

Doing this for at least thirty minutes every day will help in elevating nerve function. s

USE 15: NERVE STIMULATING BATH

This recipe uses Basil and Anise essential oil, both of which are nerve stimulating in nature. The effect of these oils is enhanced when used with Magnesium sulfate or Epsom Salt bath.

List of Ingredients:

- 1 cup Epsom Salt
- 10 drops Basil essential oil
- 5 drops Anise essential oil
- A tub of warm water

Directions:

Add all the ingredients in the tub and soak body in bath for at least 20 minutes. Repeat this a few times every week.

USE 17: NERVE BALANCING BATH

The Bergamot essential oil used in this Epsom Salt bath works wonders in balancing your nervous system.

List of Ingredients:

- 2 cups Epsom Salt

- 10 drops Bergamot essential oil
- 5 drops Lavender essential oil
- A tub of warm water

Directions:

USE 18: EPSOM SALT BATH TO RELIEVE MUSCLE STIFFNESS

Muscle stiffness can be easily relieved by mixing two cups of Epsom Salt in a tub of warm water. Add 10 drops of German Chamomile and 5 drops of Fennel oil too.

USE 19: INDIGESTION RELIEF REMEDY

Indigestion is an extremely common malady that leads to severe discomfort at times. Epsom Salt comes as a natural and handy solution in this case. A tbsp. of Epsom Salt can be dissolved in a cup of warm water to soothe an upset stomach and curb excessive acid production.

USE 20: EPSOM SALT FOR INSOMNIA

Suffering from insomnia? Epsom alt can quickly come to your rescue here. Simply add one cup of Epsom Salt to a tub full of warm water. Add a few drops of Chamomile essential oil along with 5 drops of Jasmine essential oil for added tranquility. Soak yourself in this bath for around thirty to forty minutes.

USE 21: EPSOM SALT BATH FOR A GOOD NIGHT'S SLEEP

Using Epsom Salt with essential oils derived from Valerian root can be extremely beneficial in inducing sleep. To use, just mix 1 cup Epsom Salt and 10 drops oil from the Valerian Root into a tub full of warm water. Soak for at least 40 minutes.

USE 22: EPSOM SALT TO STIMULATE BLOOD CIRCULATION

Need a relaxing blood circulation boost? Simply, take a cup of Epsom salt along with 10 drops of Rosemary essential oil, 5 drops of Eucalyptus essential oil and 4 drops of Lavender essential oil. Dissolve in a tub full of warm water and soak yourself for around 30 minutes.

Doing this every week will lead to substantial benefits.

USE 23: EPSOM SALT TO BOOST YOUR MINERAL MAGNESIUM LEVELS

If your doctor has informed you that you are deficient in magnesium, then the first thing to do is to naturally increase the quantity of magnesium in your diet. This can be done through increasing the intake of magnesium rich foods such as almonds, beans, whole grains, sesame seeds, dark chocolate, etc.

Bathing twice or thrice with any Epsom Salt recipe mentioned in the book can do the trick and help you elevate your magnesium levels.

USE 24: EPSOM SALT TO RELIEVE CONSTIPATION

Drinking a tablespoon of Epsom Salt added in a glass full of filtered water can help in relieving constipation. Make sure that you are drinking it twice a day for at least one week. You may also want to add a teaspoon of honey and juice of half a lemon into your Epsom salt water.

USE 25: EPSOM SALT FOR BLOATING

Epsom salt helps in relieving gas and bloating too. Just add a teaspoon to your ginger tea and consume twice a day. Add lime to enhance the taste.

USE 26: EPSOM SALT FOR RELIEVING GASTRITIS

Chamomile herbal tea has stomach healing properties and provides relief from gas, bloating, upset stomach and cramps. Drinking 1 tsp. of Epsom Salt in a cup of Chamomile tea twice every day can help in providing sufficient relief from bloating and gas.

USE 27: EPSOM SALT FOR GOUT

Epsom salt can work wonders in gout patients due its natural uric acid flushing properties. Take a cup of Epsom salt and add in a tub full of warm water. Also add a few drops of Peppermint essential oil and Eucalyptus essential oil into this bath. Soak yourself for at least thirty minutes. Repeat every day for at least fifteen days.

USE 28: DETOXIFICATION WITH EPSOM SALT

Try and eat only veggies and fruits on the day of your detox. Quit eating or drinking by 2:00pm and prepare to consume Epsom Salt in filtered water. To make this water and Epsom Salt mixture, mix 4 tbsp. Epsom Salt in 3 cups of water. Begin drinking this mixture at around 6:00pm. Drink in regular intervals at around 6:00pm, 8:00pm, 10:00pm and then next day at 7:00am. Eat only fruits the next day too. You may experience diarrhea. Don't worry, that is your body flushing out the toxins!

USE 29: EPSOM SALT DRINK FOR RELIEVING FEVER AND HEADACHE

Soak a washcloth in a mixture of apple cider vinegar, Epsom Salt and water and place these on the forehead and tummy of the patient. You can also wrap it around the patient's feet.

USE 30: FEVER RELIEVING EPSOM SALT BATH

An Epsom Salt warm water bath sometimes brings instantaneous fever relief. Dissolve two cups of Epsom Salt in a tub of warm water. Mix one cup of Apple Cider vinegar to this water and add five drops of Cinnamon essential oil to say goodbye to fever.

FIRST AID WITH EPSOM SALT

Epsom Salt can help you relieve some of the most common first aid fiascos. From rashes to bites to stings, this little treasure can do it all.

USE 31: HEAL YOUR SUNBURNS WITH EPSOM SALT

Spraying Epsom Salt solution over your sunburns can help in fast healing. All you need is a spray bottle filled with some clean, filtered water. Dissolve one tablespoon of Epsom salt in this water along with 10 drops of Lavender essential oil and 5 drops of Rose essential oil.

USE 32: EPSOM SALT SUNBURN HEALER

Well, this is another miraculous sunburn healing recipe involving Epsom Salt and essential oils. Just add 5 drops of Lemon essential oil along with 2 heaped tablespoons of Epsom Salt into a cup of water. Dip a clean washcloth in this and apply on impacted area once every two hours.

USE 33. RELIEVE BEE STINGS WITH EPSOM SALT

Washing the impacted area with Epsom Salt solution can help in soothing bee stings.

USE 34: EPSOM SALT BATH TO HELP IN SWELLING FROM BEE STINGS

This one is simple too. Soak yourself in any of the above mentioned Epsom Salt bath for around 30 minutes and marvel at the manner in which irritation and swelling goes away.

USE 35: EPSOM SALT AND ALOE VERA STING SOOTHER

Mix a tablespoon of Epsom Salt in a cup of warm water and boil until the water reduces to half a cup. Let the mixture cool down and add two teaspoons of pure aloe vera gel. Store in the refrigerator and apply as often as required.

USE 36: EPSOM SALT BUG BITE REMEDY

This Epsom Salt solution is superbly effective and easy to whip too. Boil a cup full of water and mix 2 teaspoons of Epsom Salt into it. Continue to stir till the solution reduces to half a cup. Let it cool down and place in the refrigerator. Apply the pasty substance directly on the impacted area.

USE 37: EPSOM SALT AND LAVENDER BUG BITE RELIEVER

Dissolve 2 tablespoons of Epsom Salt along with 10 drops of Lavender essential oil in a cup of warm water. Let it cool down and apply directly on the impacted area using a clean washcloth. Do not forget to clean and dry the area first.

USE 38: EPSOM SALT BUG BITE SOOTHER

Take 2 tablespoons of Epsom Salt and dissolve in a cup of warm water. Add 10 drops of Tea tree essential oil and 5 drops of Chamomile essential oil into the mixture and apply on impacted area using a clean washcloth.

USE 39: USING EPSOM SALT FOR TROUBLESOME SPLINTERS

Spray some Epsom Salt on that troublesome splinter and tie a clean washcloth over it. Leave it overnight. Doing this for several days can help you say bye-bye to that nasty splinter.

USE 40: USING EPSOM SALT FOR WOUNDS

Mix 5 tbsp. cold water, 2 tbsp. Epsom Salt, and 10 drops Lavender essential oil. Apply this paste over the wounds and experiencing immediate healing.

USE 41: EPSOM SALT BATH FOR INFLAMED WOUNDS

This bath soak not only helps in healing the wounds but also helps in soothing the inflammation. Just mix 2 heaped tablespoons of Epsom Salt in a tubful of warm water. Add 10 drops of Geranium essential oil to this and soak yourself for around 25 minutes. Repeat it a few times in a week to experience complete healing.

USE 42: HEALING BRUISES WITH EPSOM SALT

Mix 5 tbsp. cold water, 2 tbsp. Epsom Salt, and 10 drops Lavender essential oil. Apply this paste over the wounds and experiencing immediate healing.

USE 43: EPSOM SALT BATH FOR BRUISED SKIN

The combination of Chamomile, Lavender and magnesium sulfate make this bath soak amazingly effective for bruised and inflamed skin.

List of ingredients:

- 1 cup Epsom Salt
- 10 drops Chamomile essential oil
- 10 drops Lavender essential oil
- 1 tsp. Basil powder
- A tub full of Warm water

Directions:

Add all the ingredients in the tub and soak body in bath for at least 30 minutes.

USE 44: EPSOM SALT SOAK FOR THOSE NASTY HANGOVERS

Experiencing a hangover? Soaking in an Epsom salt bath can help you feel better instantaneously.

USE 45: EPSOM SALT FOR ALCOHOL TOXICITY

Alcohol toxicity is a result of and also leads to hangovers. Your best bet to detoxify your body and enable the magnesium ions restore their balance is by creating and soaking yourself into a luxurious Epsom Salt bath. To create this recipe, mix 2 cups of Epsom Salt in a tub full of warm water. Add 10 drops each of Lemon, Tea tree and Peppermint essential oils. Soak yourself for at least 45 minutes in order to stimulate your senses and clear your foggy mind.

USE 46: EPSOM SALT SOAK FOR THE HORRIBLE JET LAG

Jet is definitely not pretty! And that wear and tear of the mind and body is just so much bad – tiredness and fogginess are the last things you want to experience after landing at your destination. Soak yourself in an Epsom Salt bath for around thirty minutes to experience the best sleep you have ever had.

USE 47: EPSOM SALT FOR NAUSEA

Nausea is sometimes associated with jet lag and Epsom Salt comes in handy at this time too. Just use any one of the amazing bath recipes mentioned in the book and soak yourself for 20 minutes to get rid of the nausea and vomiting.

USE 48: POISON IVY EPSOM SALT COMPRESS

Mix 1 tbsp. Epsom Salt in 5 tbsp. of cold water. Add a few drops of Lavender essential oil into this paste and apply over the impacted area to get rid of the allergy.

USE 49: EPSOM SALT FOR THE ITCHING SKIN

It is often said that this miraculous salt can cure anything that itches or burns. Just create a cold compress using 2 tablespoons of Epsom Salt, 1 cup of cold water and 5 drops of Lavender oil. Apply on the impacted area several times a day to experience amazing relief.

USE 50: EPSOM SALT FOR DEEP CUTS

Do not apply Epsom Salt directly over the deep cuts. Instead soak yourself up in a bath created by diluting two cups of Epsom Salt in a tub full of warm water. Add some Lavender or Chamomile essential oil (not more than 5 drops) to experience added relief.

EPSOM SALT BATH RECIPES

Epsom Salt baths have a natural way of easing and relaxing the body, which helps in soothing the mind after a long tiring day. This chapter contains 25 amazing bath recipes that have been created using the miraculous Epsom Salt. Feel free to tweak these depending on the ingredients that you have handy.

USE 51: EPSOM SALT COCONUT BATH

This recipe can soothe your skin and help you unwind and relax after a long day. Dissolve 1 cup Epsom salt, 1 can of coconut milk, 10 drops of Lavender essential oil and 10 drops of Chamomile essential oil in a tub full of warm water. Soak yourself for around 30 minutes and experience ultimate miniaturization.

USE 52: MOISTURIZING EPSOM SALT BATH

List of Ingredients:

- ½ cup Epsom Salt
- 4 tbsp. olive oil
- Warm water (enough to fill your tub)
- 10 drops Jasmine essential oil

Directions:

Dissolve all the above mentioned ingredients in your bath tub and soak yourself for 25 minutes for nice moisturizing impact.

USE 53: SATIN SMOOTH EPSOM SALT BATH

List of Ingredients:

- ½ cup Epsom Salt
- 2 tbsp. almond oil
- A cap of almond milk
- Warm water (enough to fill your tub)
- 10 drops Chamomile essential oil

Directions:

Dissolve all the above mentioned ingredients in your bath tub and soak yourself for 40 minutes to experience the best satin smooth skin ever!

USE 54: RELIEVING HEADACHE THROUGH EPSOM SALT

This is an amazing detoxifying bath recipe, which draws out toxins and balances your skin's pH level. It works wonders on migraines and headaches too. Dissolve 1 cup Epsom Salt, 1 cup Apple cider vinegar, ½ cup Baking soda, 10 drops of Chamomile essential oil and 10 drops of Peppermint essential oil in a tub full of warm water. Soak yourself for 20 minutes.

USE 55: STRESS RELIEF EPSOM SALT BATH

Dissolve 1 cup Epsom Salt, 1 cup Baking soda, ½ cup Olive oil, 7 drops Vanilla essential oil, 2 tsp. Witch Hazel, and 10 drops Lavender essential oil in a tub full of warm water. Soak yourself for thirty minutes to experience immediate stress relief and calmness.

USE 56: MIGRAINE RELIEF EPSOM SALT BATH

List of Ingredients:

- 2 cups Epsom Salt
- Warm water (enough to fill your tub)
- 10 drops Eucalyptus essential oil
- 5 drops Rosemary essential oil

Directions:

Dissolve all the above mentioned ingredients in your bath tub and soak yourself for 20-30 minutes to experience instant relief from migraines.

USE 57: EPSOM SALT STRESS FREE BATH

The Lavender in this bath not only uplifts your mood but also provides a soothing effect. Not to mention, the headache relief from Peppermint and Rosemary essential oils.

List of Ingredients:

- 2 cups Epsom Salt
- Warm water (enough to fill your tub)
- 10 drops Peppermint essential oil
- 5 drops Rosemary essential oil
- 5 drops Lavender essential oil
- 1 teaspoon Rose essence

Directions:

Dissolve all the above mentioned ingredients in your bath tub and soak yourself for 20-30 minutes to experience instant relief from migraines.

USE 58: EPSOM SALT BODY ACHE RELIEF BATH

List of Ingredients:

- 2 cups Epsom Salt

- Warm water (enough to fill your tub)
- 10 drops Eucalyptus essential oil
- 5 drops Roman Chamomile essential oil
- 5 drops Lavender essential oil

Directions:

Dissolve all the above mentioned ingredients in your bath tub and soak yourself for around 25 minutes to experience instant relief from migraines.

USE 59: EPSOM SALT BATH TO HEAL NEURALGIA

Neuralgia can be really painful and Epsom Salt can work wonders there as well. Just mix two cups of Epsom Salt in tub full of warm water. Add 5 drops of Helichrysum essential oil and 10 drops of Peppermint essential oil to this mixture. Soak yourself for around 15 minutes. You can increase the duration to 30 minutes gradually. Also increase the quantity of Epsom Salt to 3 cups gradually. Soak yourself in this bath at least three times in a week to witness amazing results.

USE 60: EPSOM SALT BATH TO HEAL NEUROPATHY

The tingling sensation in hands and feet can sometimes worsen into Carpal Tunnel or other complications. Luckily, Epsom Salt comes as your trusted companion in this case too!

List of Ingredients:

- 2 cups Epsom Salt
- Warm water (enough to fill your tub)
- 10 drops Patchouli essential oil
- 5 drops Tangerine essential oil
- 5 drops Ylang Ylang essential oil

Directions:

Dissolve all the above mentioned ingredients in your bath tub and soak yourself for around 30 minutes to experience relief from the tingling sensation. Repeat this process a few times each week.

USE 61: ESSENTIAL OIL BATH TO TREAT INSOMNIA

2 cups Epsom salt is mixed with 10 drops of roman Chamomile oil and 5 drops of Ylang Ylang oil and dissolved into a tubful of warm water. Soak yourself in this bath for 20 minutes every night to experience the most peaceful sleep ever.

USE 62: GENERAL WELL BEING BATH SALT

Dissolve 2 cups Epsom Salt, 1 cup Olive oil, 10 drops Eucalyptus oil and 10 drops Peppermint oil in a tub full of warm water and soak yourself for around 20 minutes to elevate general well-being.

USE 63: EPSOM SALT BATH TO RECLAIM YOUR SINUSES

List of Ingredients:

- 2 cups Epsom Salt
- Warm water (enough to fill your tub)
- 10 drops Clove oil
- 2 drops Peppermint essential oil

Directions:

Dissolve all the above mentioned ingredients in your bath tub and soak yourself for around 25 minutes to clear those blocked nasal passages and relieve all respiratory inflammation.

USE 64: EPSOM OIL BATH FOR VARICOSE VEINS

A simple bath soak every day can help you get rid of varicose veins naturally. Just take 2 cups of Epsom Salt and dissolve in a tub of warm water. Soak for at least 20 minutes, preferably twice every day.

USE 65: EPSOM OIL ANTI-INFLAMMATORY AND MOISTURIZING BODY BATH

List of Ingredients:

- 2 cups Epsom Salt
- Warm water (enough to fill your tub)
- 10 drops Orange oil
- 10 drops Helichrysum essential oil
- 1 cup coconut milk
- 2 tbsp. olive oil

Directions:

Dissolve all the above mentioned ingredients in your bath tub and soak yourself for at least 45 minutes three times in a week.

USE 66: EPSOM OIL BATH SALT FOR AGELESS SKIN

Take 2 cups of Epsom Salt and dissolve in a tub full of warm water. Dissolve 10 drops of Neroli essential oil and 5 drops of Myrrh essential oil in this water.

Soak yourself for atleast 20 minutes every day to reveal fresh, wrinkle free ageless skin.

USE 67: EPSOM SALT ANTI-WRINKLE BATH

Mix 1 cup Epsom Salt with 10 drops each of Ylang Ylang, Patchouli, Tea tree and Lavender essential oil. Shake it properly and dissolve in a tub full of warm water.

Soak yourself for at least 40 minutes every alternate day.

USE 68: EPSOM SALT BATH SALT FOR HAY FEVER

Mix 2 cups of Epsom salt in a tub of warm water. Add 10 drops of Tea tree essential oil and 5 drops of Roman Chamomile essential oil to this water and soak yourself for around 15-20 minutes twice a day.

USE 69: EPSOM SALT BATH FOR CLEAR SKIN

Mix a cup of Epsom Salt with 5 drops each of Bergamot, Tea Tree and Oregano essential oil. Dissolve in a tub of warm water and soak yourself for around 40 minutes. Repeat thrice a week for amazing, clear, acne free skin.

USE 70: EPSOM SALT TO TREAT ACNE SCARS

Dissolve a cup of Epsom Salt and 5 drops each of Frankincense, Carrot seed and Lavender oil into a tub full of warm water and soak yourself up for 20 minutes each day. Doing this for fifteen to twenty days can help in completely healing the acne scars.

USE 71: EPSOM SALT FOR SKIN BRIGHTENING

A cup of Epsom Salt, 5 drops of Jasmine, Lemon and 3Lavender essential oils combined with a tub of warm water is the perfect recipe to brighten your skin. Soak every day for fifteen minutes. Visible results can be seen in 15-20 days.

USE 72: EPSOM SALT TO CURE COLD SORES

10 drops of Tea tree essential oil, 5 drops of Sage essential oil, 5 drops of Sandalwood essential oil and 1 cup of Epsom Salt dissolved in a tub of warm water can help in curing cold sores.

USE 73: EPSOM SALT BATH FOR MOOD SWINGS

This one is extremely effective in PMS, depression and other mood swings. Immerse yourself in the luxury of Epsom Salt bath created by dissolving 2 cups Epsom Salt in 1 tub full of warm water with 10 drops of Rose Otto essential oil and 5 drops of Jasmine essential oil.

USE 74: ENERGIZING EPSOM SALT BATH BLEND

List of Ingredients:

- 2 cups Epsom Salt
- Warm water (enough to fill your tub)
- 10 drops Orange oil
- 10 drops Lemon essential oil
- 5 drops Bergamot essential oil

Directions:

Dissolve all the above mentioned ingredients in your bath tub and soak yourself for at least 20 minutes to regain the lost energy.

USE 75: ANXIETY RELIEF EPSOM SALT BATH BLEND

Mix 10 drops of Lavender essential oil, 5 drops of Clary Sage essential and 2 cups Epsom Salt in a tub full of warm water. Soak yourself in this water for 20 minutes to experience relief from anxiety and depression.

BEAUTY BENEFITS OF EPSOM SALT

The Epsom Salt beauty recipes mentioned in this chapter will ensure that your exterior is as healthful as your interior.

USE 76: EPSOM SALT EXFOLIATING SCRUB

Prepare your very own exfoliating scrub using 2 cups Epsom Salt, 4 tbsp. olive oil, juice of one medium sized lemon, 1 tbsp. basil leaf powder and 1 tbsp. oatmeal powder. Use this one of twice a week dry or in shower.

USE 77: EPSOM SALT SKIN SOOTHING SCRUB

This is prepared by mixing 1 cup Epsom Salt, 2 tbsp. Almond oil, juice of half medium sized lemon and a handful of dried rosemary leaves. Use twice a week for best results.

USE 78: EPSOM SALT ANTI ACNE SCRUB

To prepare this, mix 1 cup of Epsom Salt with 3 tbsp. of coconut oil and 5 drops of Carrot Seed oil. Use every day to notice visible reduction in acne and scars.

USE 79: EPSOM SALT SCRUB FOR FAIRNESS.

A simple Epsom Salt fairness scrub can be made by mixing a cup of Epsom Salt with 10 drops of Lemon essential oil and a tbsp. Almond oil. You must use it every day to notice visible results within 10-15 days.

USE 80: EPSOM SALT ANTI-WRINKLE SCRUB

To prepare this, mix a cup of Epsom Salt with two tablespoons of sweet almond oil and 10 drops of Frankincense essential oil. Use in shower every day.

USE 81: EPSOM SALT FACIAL CLEANSER

Mix Epsom Salt with a pinch of cinnamon and a tbsp. of coconut oil. Use it as a purifying natural cleanser.

USE 82: EPSOM SALT BASED BODY BUTTER

Mix 1 cup of Epsom Salt with 2 tbsp. of boiling water. Combine 2 tbsp. beeswax, 3 tbsp. of Shea butter, ¼ cup of olive oil and ½ cup of sweet almond oil in a jar and place this jar in a pan with water. Place this pan over medium heat and wait until the mixture melts. Blend the oil mixture and slowly add the Epsom salt mix. Now, place in the fridge to get the consistency of body butter. Apply as and when required.

USE 83: EPSOM SALT SATIN SMOOTH BODY BUTTER

Mix 1 cup of Epsom Salt with 2 tbsp. of boiling water. Combine 2 tbsp. beeswax, 3 tbsp. of Cocoa butter and ½ cup of almond oil in a jar and place this jar in a pan with water. Place this pan over medium heat and wait until the mixture melts. Blend the oil mixture and slowly add the Epsom salt mix. Now, place in the fridge to get the consistency of body butter. Apply as and when required.

USE 84: ANTI BLEMISH BODY BUTTER USING EPSOM SALT

Mix 1 cup of Epsom Salt with 2 tbsp. of boiling water. Combine 2 tbsp. beeswax, 3 tbsp. of Shea butter, ½ cup of almond oil, 20 drops of Lemon essential oil, 10 drops of Frankincense essential oil and ¼ cup of coconut oil in a jar and place this jar in a pan with water. Place this pan over medium heat and wait until the mixture melts. Blend the oil mixture and slowly add the Epsom salt mix. Now, place in the fridge to get the consistency of body butter. Apply as and when required.

USE 85: VITAMIN E RICH EPSOM SALT BODY BUTTER

This body butter is offer amazing benefits of vitamin E along with the mineral magnesium. Mix 1 cup of Epsom Salt with 2 tbsp. of boiling water. Combine 1 cup cocoa butter and 1 cup extra virgin olive oil a jar and place this jar in a pan with water. Place this pan over medium heat and wait until the mixture melts. Now, puncture 6 capsules of vitamin E and add to the blend. Next, add the Epsom salt mix. Now, place in the fridge to get the consistency of body butter. Apply as frequently as required.

USE 86: EPSOM SALT BODY BRONZING BODY BUTTER

Nutmeg, cinnamon and cacao powder — whipped together along with Epsom Salt into a luxuriously aromatic creamy spread – wow! What a treat! To prepare, gently melt 1 cup Shea butter in a pan using the double boiler method. Next, pour 1 cup coconut oil into this and continue to stir until blended. Let the mixture cool down and add ¼ cup of almond oil, 1 tbsp. ground nutmeg, 1 tbsp. ground cinnamon and 1 tbsp. cacao powder into the mixture. Now, add 1 cup of Epsom Salt and place this mixture in the refrigerator. Whip it after 20 minutes and use as frequently as desired.

USE 87: DOUBLE MAGNESIUM MAGIC BODY BUTTER

Take ½ cup magnesium flakes in a container and pour around ½ cup of boiling water over them. Keep stirring until they are completely dissolved and a thick liquid is formed. Add 1 cup Epsom Salt to this mixture and set aside to cool.

Now, take 1 cup Shea butter, 4 tbsp. beeswax and 1 cup coconut oil in a separate pan and mix these using the double boiler method. Add the magnesium mixture and let it cool. Allow it to set in the refrigerator.

USE 88: SUPER LUSCIOUS AND NOURISHING EPSOM SALT BODY BUTTER

This one is prepared using 1 cup Epsom Salt, 1 cup Shea butter, 1 cup coconut oil, 4 tbsp. Jojoba oil and 20 drops of Rose essential oil.

Truly magical and divine!

USE 89: BYE BYE TO BLEMISHES WITH EPSOM SALT

Boil a cup of water and add 3 drops iodine along with 10 drops of Rose essential oil, 5 drops of Lavender essential oil and 1 tbsp. of Epsom Salt into it. Stir till mixed well. Allow to cool and pack in an airtight container to be stored in the refrigerator. Apply frequently over blemishes. Keep for fifteen minutes and wash with cold water.

USE 90: EPSOM SALT ANTI MARKS OINTMENT

Boil a cup of water and add a few basil leaves into it along with 1 tbsp. of Epsom Salt. Continue to stir till mixed well and until the water reduces to half a cup. Allow to cool and pack in an airtight container to be stored in the refrigerator. Use a cotton swab to apply over blemishes, let it sit for 10 minutes and rinse off with cold water.

USE 91: EPSOM SALT ANTI BLACKHEADS OINTMENT

A cup of Epsom Salt is added to 2 cups of water and boiled until a pasty consistency is achieved. 2 tbsp. of cucumber juice is added to this along with 10 drops of Lemon essential oil. This can be stored in the refrigerator and used thrice a day for visible results.

USE 92: EPSOM SALT DARK CIRCLES OINTMENT

Boil a cup of water and add 2 tbsp. Epsom Salt into it. Next, add some lemon juice and 5 drops of lime essential oil into this. Store it in an airtight container once it cools down and apply as frequently as you would like.

USE 93: EPSOM SALT OINTMENT FOR DRY AND FLAKY SKIN

Boil a cup of water and add a 2 tbsp. olive oil into it along with 1 tbsp. of Epsom Salt. Continue to stir till mixed well and until the water reduces to half a cup. Add 2 tbsp. coconut milk to this mixture and allow it to cool. Pack in an airtight container and store in the refrigerator. Use a cotton swab to apply over dry skin, let it sit for 10 minutes and rinse off with cold water.

USE 94: EPSOM SALT OINTMENT FOR PUFFY EYES

Boil a cup of water and add a 2 tbsp. extra virgin coconut oil into it along with 1 tbsp. of Epsom Salt. Continue to stir till mixed well and until the water reduces to half a cup. Add 2 tbsp. of cucumber juice to this mixture and allow it to cool. Pack in an airtight container and store in the refrigerator. Use a cotton swab to apply under the eye area, let it sit for 10 minutes and rinse off with cold water.

USE 95: EPSOM SALT OINTMENT FOR WRINKLED HANDS

Boil a cup of water and add a 2 tbsp. of sweet almond oil into it along with 1 tbsp. of Epsom Salt. Continue to stir till mixed well and until the water reduces to half a cup. Add ½ cup of coconut milk to this mixture and allow it to cool. Pack in an airtight container and store in the refrigerator. Use it as often as possible to nourish your hands.

USE 96: EPSOM SALT SCRUB FOR CHAPPED LIPS

This is an extremely simple recipe that helps in getting rid of dry, flaky, unsightly lips. Combine a teaspoon of maple syrup, 10 drops rose essential oil and a tablespoon of Epsom Salt. Apply over your dry lips to experience immediate moisture and glow!

USE 97: EPSOM SALT SCRUB FOR DRY HEELS

Get an instant pedicure at home using Epsom Salt. Dip your feet in a tub of warm water mixed with 1 tbsp. Epsom Salt. Pat dry using a towel and apply the Epsom salt ointments for wrinkled hands (recipe above) over the heels too!

USE 98: EPSOM SALT FOR ORAL HYGIENE

Gargle with a tablespoon of Epsom Salt added in a cup of warm water. Add a dash of lemon juice for flavor.

USE 99: EPSOM SALT RINSE FOR ORAL ULCERS

Oral ulcers can be extremely painful. Use 2 tbsp. Epsom Salt dissolved in a cup of room temperature water infused with a tbsp. of basil leaves to experience relief from oral ulcers.

USE 100: EPSOM SALT RISE TO PURIFY THE SCALP

Combine 2 tbsp. Epsom Salt, 1 cup hot water and ½ cup lemon juice. Allow it to cool for some time and apply to dampened scalp. Let it soak for around 10 minutes. Rinse thoroughly followed by your regular shampoo routine.

USE 101: EPSOM SALT HAIR MASK

Combine 1 cup Epsom Salt, 1 cup warm water, ½ cup lemon juice, 3 tbsp. coconut oil and 10 drops of Jasmine essential oil. Allow it to cool and apply over dampened scalp. Leave on for thirty minutes and rinse with your regular shampoo.

USE 102: EPSOM SALT NATURAL HAIR CONDITIONER

Combine 2 tbsp. sweet almond oil with 2 tbsp. Epsom Salt and 1 tbsp. baking soda. Apply like your regular conditioner and notice results within a few weeks.

USE 103: EPSOM SALT VOLUMIZING CONDITIONER

Combine 2 tbsp. Epsom Salt with 2 tbsp. Extra virgin coconut oil and use like your regular conditioner. Noticeable results will be visible in a few weeks.

USE 104: EPSOM SALT FOOT SOAK

Combine 1 cup Epsom Salt, 1 foot tub of warm water, 2 tbsp. lemon juice, ½ cup Apple cider vinegar and few drops of Lavender essential oil. Soak feet for at least thirty minutes. Repeat few times in a week.

USE 105: EPSOM SALT EYE COMPRESS

Mix 3 tbsp. Epsom Salt in 3 tbsp. hot water. Let the mixture cool down and then add some cucumber juice into it. Dip a clean washcloth and place over closed eyes for a few minutes. Repeat morning and evening for best results. !

USE 106: EPSOM SALT INFUSED SHAMPOO

Craving for extra nourishment for your hair? Mix 1 tbsp. Epsom Salt into your regular shampoo to witness some amazing nourishment and deep cleansing.

USE 107: EPSOM SALT FACE MASK FOR ACNE PRONE SKIN

Mix 1 tbsp. honey, 1 tbsp. Epsom Salt, 1 tsp. baking soda and juice of half a lemon to prepare the best face mask to treat your acne.

USE 108: EPSOM SALT FACE MASK FOR BEAUTIFUL SKIN

Mix a tablespoon of Epsom Salt with 1 tablespoon of Apple cider vinegar and ½ tablespoon honey. Apply on face, keep for 20 minutes and rinse.

USE 109: EPSOM SALT MASK FOR DRY SKIN

Blend 1 cup grated carrot, 1 cup Epsom Salt and 1 cup mayonnaise. Spread over damp skin, wait for ten minutes and remove.

USE 110: EPSOM SALT MASK FOR OILY SKIN

Blend 1 egg, 2 tbsp. Epsom Salt, 1 tbsp. non-fat dry milk and juice of 1 lemon. Apply to damp skin, wait for five minutes and rinse off.

USE 111: EPSOM SALT HAIRSPRAY REMOVER

Take a gallon of water and add one cup of Epsom Salt into it. Also add 1 cup lemon juice and let this mixture infuse overnight. The next morning, apply prior to your shampoo ritual and notice the hairspray gone!

USE 112: EPSOM SALT WHITENING TOOTHPASTE

Mix 1 tbsp. Epsom Salt with a little hydrogen peroxide. Brush your teeth with this mixture. Although it tastes terrible, it promises amazing benefits.

USING EPSOM SALT FOR WEIGHT LOSS

Bathing in a warm Epsom Salt soak helps in flushing out the toxins, which in turn leads to weight loss.

USE 113: EPSOM SALT SCRUB TO TREAT CELLULITE

Mix 4 tbsp. Honey, 2 tbsp. Epsom Salt, 2 tbsp. Brown Sugar and 1 tbsp. lemon juice. Massage into the problems areas, leave for two minutes and rinse with warm water.

USE 114: EPSOM SALT SOAK FOR RAPID WEIGHT LOSS

Add 1 cup Epsom Salt, 1 cup Apple cider vinegar, 1 tbsp. ginger powder, and 10 drops grapefruit essential oil into a tubful of warm water. Soak for 20 minutes.

USE 115: 'FIT INTO SKINNY JEANS' EPSOM SALT SOAK

Want a temporary and quick fix 'fit into the skinny jeans' remedy? Just soak yourself into a warm water tub infused with 2 cups of Epsom Salt for around 10 minutes. You will be pleasantly surprised by the instant results.

USE 120: SPECIAL EPSOM SALT RAPID WEIGHT LOSS BATH

Mix 2 cups Epsom Salt and 1 cup Baking soda into a tub full of warm water. Soak yourself in this bath for at least 25 minutes every day. If you cannot do every day, try every alternate day in order to achieve consistent and visible weight loss.

USE 121: EPSOM SALT AND ACV WEIGHT LOSS BATH

Epsom Salt and ACV can work wonders for your weight loss when used together. Dissolve 1 cup Epsom Salt and 1 cup ACV in a tub full of warm water. Soak yourself for 20 minutes every day to experience some amazing long term inch loss.

USE 122: EPSOM SALT ANTI BLOATING BATH

Add 1 cup Epsom Salt, 1 tbsp. dried ginger and 10 drops of Eucalyptus essential oil into a tub full of warm water. Soak yourself for at least 20 minutes three times a week.

USE 123: EPSOM SALT WEIGHT LOSS DRINK

Mix 1 tbsp. Epsom Salt and 1 gm. Cumin powder into a glass of warm water. Drink slowly followed by another glass of normal, filtered water. Visible results can be seen in thirty days or less.

USE 124: EPSOM SALT WEIGHT LOSS AID

You can create your own mild Epsom Salt induced water by mixing 1 tbsp. Epsom Salt in 1 liter of water. Sip throughout the day.

USE 125: EPSOM SALT ANTI BLOATING DRINK

Mix 1 tbsp. Epsom Salt, 1 tsp. grated ginger and 1 tsp. ACV in a glass full of water. Drink slowly for three consecutive days. Give a gap of three days and drink again for three days. Continue this for as long as you can.

EPSOM SALT TO NOURISH YOUR GARDEN

Just as Epsom Salt is great for the body and mind, it can work wonders for nourishing your plants too.

USE 126: EPSOM SALT AS FERTILIZER

Dilute 5 tbsp. Epsom Salt per 1 gallon of water. Allow the mixture to dissolve and transfer into a spray bottle. Spritz directly on to your plants once per month in replacement of regular watering.

USE 127: HEALTHY PEPPERS, TOMATOES AND ROSES

Mix 1 tbsp. Epsom Salt in a gallon of water. Spray on surrounding soil every few weeks.

USE 128: EPSOM SALT DIRECT APPLICATION FOR TOMATOES AND PEPPERS

Mix 2 tbsp. Epsom Salt in half a bucket of water. Scoop a small handful and sprinkle it at the base of your plants.

USE 129: EPSOM SALT INSECT AND PEST REPELLANT

Just put some Epsom salt into areas frequented by pests and get pleasantly surprised with the amazing difference.

USE 130: EPSOM SALT FERTILIZER FOR FRUIT TREES

Mixing Epsom Salt in the soil near your fruits will do the trick here.

USE 131: EPSOM SALT SPRAY FOR GREENER GRASS

Spray Epsom Salt over your grass every three months and experience the best lawns ever.

USE 132: LUSCIOUS LAWNS USING EPSOM SALT

You can even combine Epsom salt with water and spray over your grass. I bet, you will be amazed at the quality of your lawns.

USE 133: EPSOM SALT TO DEODORIZE COMPOST

Just add some Epsom Salt into your compost and experience complete deodorization.

USE 134: EPSOM SALT TO REMOVE STUMPS

Epsom Salt can be poured over stumps to remove them too.

USE 135: EPSOM SALT FOR BETTER FLOWERING

Addition of Epsom Salt into the garden can help in better flowering.

USE 136: EPSOM SALT FOR BETTER NUTRIENT ABSORPTION

Addition of Epsom Salt into the soil can help plants take up vital nutrients, eliminating the need for chemical fertilizers.

USE 137: EPSOM SAT TO PREVENT LEAF CURLING

Application of Epsom Salt near the base of leaves will prevent them from curling.

USE 138: EPSOM SALT TO COUNTER TRANSPLANT SHOCK

Roots can be damaged and transplant shock can occur when you move plants from one place to another. After planting, water the plants with 1 gallon of water mixed with 1 tbsp. Epsom Salt.

USE 139: EPSOM SALT FOR PALM TREES FRIZZLE TOP

Magnesium deficiency in palms can lead to frizzle tops. Apply Epsom Salt around the base and drench the leaves and crown with a liquid mixture of 1 tbsp. to 1 gallon of water.

USE 140: EPSOM SALT WEED KILLER

Mix 2 cups Epsom Salt with 1 gallon of vinegar. Add a liquid dish soap into the mixture and put in a spray bottle. Then spray over weeds, carefully avoiding leaves and other plants. This will kill the weeds in the most efficient way.

EPSOM SALT FOR HOUSEHOLD USE

Finally, it is time to discover the wonderful uses of Epsom Salt in your home.

USE 141: EPSOM SALT CLEANER FOR TILES

Combine 1 cup Epsom Salt, 1 cup baking soda and ½ cup vinegar. Scrub over tiles using clockwise motion. Rinse thoroughly.

USE 142: POT AND PAN CLEANER

You can clean your pots and pans with Epsom salt too.

USE 143: EPSOM SALT HOUSE PLANT REFRESHER

Spraying Epsom Salt over house plants can help in maintenance.

USE 144: EPSOM SALT CARPET CLEANER

A mixture of Epsom Salt and water works well when it comes to cleaning carpets and rugs.

USE 145: EPSOM SALT RUST REMOVERS

A combination of Epsom Salt, water and lemon juice can be used to scrub off the rust.

USE 146: EPSOM SALT FABRIC SOFTENER

Add ½ tablespoon Epsom Salt and 10 drops of Jasmine essential oil to your favorite laundry cleaner and drool over the softness of your clothes.

USE 147: EPSOM SALT TO FILL HOLES IN THE WALL

A thick paste of Epsom Salt can help in filling the holes in the wall

USE 148: EPSOM SALT WASHING MACHINE CLEANSER

A mixture of Epsom Salt and white vinegar can be used to clean washing machines too.

USE 149: REGENERATING YOUR CAR BATTERY

Dissolve about an ounce of Epsom Salt in warm water and add to each battery cell.

USE 150: FROST YOUR WINDOWS FOR CHRISTMAS

Dreaming of a white Christmas and the weather doesn't seem to cooperate? Well, Epsom salt can come to your rescue here too. Mix Epsom Salt with stale bear until it stops dissolving. Apply this mixture to your windows with a sponge. The windows look frosted once the mixture dries.

CONCLUSION

You have now discovered the numerous ways Epsom Salt can be incorporated into your daily life and routine. Thank you for purchasing this book and joining me in the journey to explore and incorporate natural and effective ingredients for a variety of everyday tasks. I hope that you will found these tips, and recipes to be useful for your health and home. Wishing you much success!

*Bonus Book 1

HOW TO START A PROFITABLE BLOG

A Guide To Create Content That Rocks, Build Traffic, And Turn Your Blogging Passion Into Profit (Blog Mastermind Booklets)

Contents

Introduction

I want to thank you and congratulate you for downloading the book, *"How to Start A Profitable Blog: A Guide To Create Content That Rocks, Build Traffic, And Turn Your Blogging Passion Into Profit (Blog Mastermind Booklets)*.

This book contains valuable information on how to kick start your income stream with a blog. After reading this book, you should have the understandings of what a blog is, and how to fully optimize your blog online. Keep in mind, when creating your blog, to focus on creating value, instead of just trying to make money. Creating value is important, because in order for you to get what you want, you have to first give others what they want. And know, that when your passive income exceeds your expenses, that is when you'll be financially free to replace your day job for life.

The phrase financial freedom includes the word financial, but it also includes the word freedom: Freedom to explore the blessings that surround us. Freedom to help ourselves so that we can help others. Freedom to live the life we choose to lead, instead of having to live the life that was chosen for us.

Thanks again for downloading this book, I hope it inspires you to create, and to follow your dreams.

CHAPTER ONE: GETTING STARTED WITH BLOGGING

"Self expression has become the new entertainment"
– Arianna Huffington

Almost everybody is a blogger these days – irrespective of the fact whether they realize it or not.

Have you ever written something on Facebook and received a few likes and may be some comments as well?

Awesome! You are a blogger.

Did you ever tweet a short sentence on Twitter?

Congratulations! You are a micro blogger!

How about uploading a YouTube video where you can obtain a few subscribers and prompt a few comments?

Well – you have begun videoblogging too!

Blogging leads to an outburst of expression and creativity, which in turn opens up digital doors for an expert who has till now been invisible.

And the best part – you do not have to wait for twenty five long years in order to be declared as an expert in a particular field. *Just declare yourself and publish*.

Isn't it easy?

Let us first try and understand the whole concept – **what is a blog and why so much hype around blogging**?

A blog is short for Web log. In layman terms, it is just a website with entries listed in a reverse chronological order. The original idea behind the creation of a blog was to create an online diary or journal that could be updated every day.

During the past few years, a number of software companies have developed platforms that have made the process of blogging extremely simple – you write your story, click 'submit,' and voila – it shows on your blog for the world to take notice of you and your brand.

But I am not a techie?

No problem. You don't worry on that front since most bloggers do not understand any programming language and the companies that have developed these platforms acknowledge that.

Starting a blog can be one of the simplest processes to start a website. It is quick to set up and sometimes completely free.

Even if there are steps to follow, they are extremely simple and then, there are plenty of resources to help you along the way.

Here are some interesting facts about blogs:

- Every half a second – a new blog is created somewhere in the world.
- This signifies an addition of 172,800 blogs to the internet every day.
- As on date, there are 152 million blogs on the internet.

Still thinking about the process? Well, if there are so many blog, the process just cannot be difficult.

THE COSTS INVOLVED

A number of services are available in order to empower you to start your blog – and that too for free. If you are simply going to be experimenting with the entire process of blogging, I would recommend a free service in order to first understand the process.

Once you get your feet wet and decide to stick with it and eventually make money with your blog, you can upgrade yourself to a self-hosted blog.

Getting a self-hosted blog is inexpensive – the domain name costs around $10 per year and webhosting is approximately a few bucks every month.

THE BLOGGING PLATFORMS

Well, if you are looking at creating a great blog and generating some passive income from it too, then I would suggest that you do not waste time with Blogger.com or WordPress.com . You will eventually want to change it – the sooner you do, the better it is for your blog.

I personally recommend being self-hosted on WordPress.org - this is more or less the industry standard today. You would need to pay a few dollars a month for hosting, but the income that you will generate eventually makes up for the expenses. Try and pick up a .com name that matches your site name.

Once you set up your blog on WordPress, you begin the process of content creation. This is in fact the most critical part of your blog. Remember, people will come for killer content – they definitely may get impressed by the pretty design or layout, however, that is not something that will get them back – only killer content can get them back and even generate some referrals.

The next thing that you need is an amazing layout and design. I recommend that you hire someone to help you with this process (unless, of course you are a graphic designer yourself). An experienced designer can help you create a layout that becomes a visual representation of your content, your feelings, your personality, and yourself!

WHAT SHOULD YOU WRITE ABOUT?

Well, the best thing to begin with is to create amazing, compelling content – content that brings your readers back to your blog. This implies that your blog has to be truly awesome. The key here is to discover what 'awesome' means to you. Everyone has a passion – something that they are too good at, something that they can share and that their readers can learn from. Discover your true passion and decide on a topic. Remember, everything that you publish should be meaningful – there has to be a definite intention behind whatever you decide to publish. The content has to be amazing and should add value to the readers.

Here are some questions that you can ask yourself before deciding on the subject for your blog:

- What is it that you love to do most?
- What are the things that you are really passionate about?

- What are the topics that people ask you for advice?
- What are the subjects that you are naturally drawn towards?
- What subjects do you love to read most?
- What gets you so fired up that you can't stop talking about?

You must also have a clear plan on what you want to write about. This will include a main topic, then a few sub topics and then a few categories beneath each subtopic.

Let us take an example here – If your main topic is 'Living well on a budget,' your sub-topics could be 'Using coupons to your advantage,' 'DIY recipes', 'Tips to declutter your home,' 'Ideas to save money during the holiday season,' etc. Now, here the main theme is pretty broad and includes a couple of sub themes – however, it does not include everything. Therefore, the readers of the blog are aware of what to expect when they visit the blog.

Now, imagine this blog owner starting with movie reviews and then reviews of latest makeup and gadgets and then reviews of various restaurants in the town. This will only confuse the reader and they will think that the blog owner does not understand their content too well.

Therefore, *it is important to have a clear structure and plan in place.*

Readers always crave authenticity – don't hold things back, be authentic and give everything that you have got. Just focus on making your blog awesome.

Go through the blogs that you love but never try and BE those blogs. *Be your own voice – be authentic – be passionate – focus on your individual strengths that can make your readers life awesome*.

So, let us review the action items from this chapter:

- Spend some time with yourself, trying to discover your passion which will translate into your blog's main theme, sub theme and sub topics.
- Pick up a great blog name and set up a self-hosted blog on WordPress.org
- If you are not a graphic designer, get professional help with the layout and design.
- Create compelling content that is truly awesome and adds value to your readers.

CHAPTER TWO: CREATING CONTENT THAT ROCKS

Alright, for a moment – let us think about your favorite blog. *Is there a blog that you are always dying to read – that you check out even before a new post is released?*

Now, take a moment to think about the things that you love in this blog.

- Does this blog have a cool theme?
- Do you love the font that they use?
- Is it their choice of colors?
- Do you like the fact that they have over five thousand Facebook followers?

Well, the blog may have all of that, but chances are that you are solely captivated by the content. You love to read stuff that you can relate to, don't you? You love to read stuff that adds value. You love to read through those mouth-watering recipes or DIY household projects and can't wait to try some yourself. You love commenting on the blog post and sharing your results. In fact, you have even accepted the thirty days de-clutter challenge and are fully motivated to share your results.

In simple language, your favorite blog rocks because it contains content that rocks!

Try and create content that can add value, that you are passionate about and that your readers can benefit from.

My next suggestion for you is to create a **calendar of events** for your blog.

But, I can only write when I am in a mood!

True, most bloggers start like that. They decide to write only if they are in a mood to write. Mostly, the result is an unorganized blog where readers do not know what to expect and when to expect.

My suggestion here is that if you are serious about blogging and looking to earn some money through your passion, you must create a calendar of events. It could be a simple word or excel document where you mention about what you would post every day.

Here is an example:

September 2015

Week one:

- Monday: Monday morning mantra – simple 30 minute yoga for the week
- Tuesday: Tuesday healthy tips – Healthy tips from the kitchen
- Wednesday: Wednesday Recipe – Healthy Wednesday recipe – banana oatmeal with kale and orange smoothie
- Thursday: Things no one will tell you about hormones and PMS (yes, it is impacting your relationships but not anymore!)
- Friday: Friday family fun: Fun exercises for the whole family
- Saturday: Tips to encourage your kids towards healthy eating (bonus: healthy blueberry pie recipe)
- Sunday: no post

You could even use different colored highlighters to ensure that posts that are in progress stand out and posts that have been completed and posted are hidden or highlighted in a different color. I like to use a green highlighter for posts that are in progress, a red highlighter for posts that are due but not started and a blue highlighter for posts that have been completed.

Ideally, your calendar must be planned at least two months in advance and posts should be written at least a fortnight in advance. It may be necessary to shuffle things up a little, however, make sure to stick to the plan as much as possible.

Adequate planning can ensure that you are sticking to the plan even when on a break. Imagine, how cool it would be to post something on your blog as you holiday with family on the mountains or at the beach. All you need to do is pick up a post that you have already written and plug it in there.

Now, you may think that it is going to be difficult to come up with two months of awesome, brand new content. Well, the key here is **effective brainstorming**. Every week, you must set aside some time for yourself. This is the time when you will be at your peak capacity. Keep loads of colored sticky notes on a table and write down your blog sub categories. Now, for the next half an hour, just think about what your readers would want to see from you in the next fifteen days or so. Write down whatever comes into your mind. If you cannot think about anything for a particular category, leave it blank and come back to it later.

Now, take all your sticky notes and get organized. Use the next half an hour to convert these ideas into catchy titles for your blogpost.

Remember, this method of brainstorming is not cast in stone. You may like to brainstorm as you clean the house or every day in the shower. That is totally your call. Decide on what works best for you and work accordingly.

TIPS TO WRITING A GREAT BLOG POST

Let me say this upfront – if you dislike writing, then probably blogging is not meant for you. In order to write a blog post, you need to practice the discipline of writing. Decide on a time every day and force yourself to write a certain number of words – I like to write around a 1,000 words at a time. This makes two blog posts a day – one in the morning and one in the evening. Depending on your goals, you could decide on your daily target and make sure that you meet it – practicing to write a certain number of words every day will greatly elevate your writing style.

A fantastic blog post means greater traffic on your blog, more pins on Pinterest, more Facebook shares and more tweets. *The impact of all this*?

All these help your blog to grow.

Here are some of the things that you must do as you write a blog post:

Your post must make a clear point: Sometimes, writers keep writing about a number of things and towards the end, the reader gets lost – thinking – "*well, what was he really trying to say*?" To maintain the interest of your readers, write blog posts that make a point. These posts can be easily summarized in one sentence.

Your post must be visually appealing: You must ensure that your blog posts carry amazing images to go with them. With the advent of Pinterest, this is an important factor for all your posts.

Your posts must teach ONE simple lesson: Now, I am not trying to discourage you from writing about complicated projects and ideas. However, with time I have realized that you receive maximum traffic on posts that are really simple – just one simple lesson is all that people want to read through one post.

Your posts must evoke an emotional response: Most posts that generate traffic are the ones that make people feel a certain way – they could make you happy, sad, angry, empathetic, grateful or encouraged. Make sure that people are able to relate to what you write and your post generates an emotional response.

Your posts make your readers go WOW: It is better to share one blog post that generates a WOW response than post many that do not stir up any feelings or conversations. Write about things that you are passionate about and that your readers can't help but pay attention to – *they must be able to stop everything and just focus on your post*.

Your posts should encourage and empower your readers: Imagine sharing a really nice picture with a really complicated recipe. Since the picture is nice, it definitely attracts attention. But the recipe? Well, your readers lose interest the moment they begin reading it. It is too complicated to follow and they cannot relate to it. *They don't see themselves preparing that dish!*

How about including some tips that can make the recipe simple? You could even write about the difficulties that you faced and the steps that you took in in order to overcome those.

Your readers have to feel that they CAN do it too!

<u>Your posts must be unique and interesting</u>: Your posts must have something amazing, new and interesting to say. Ideally, after reading your post your readers must be able to look at a problem in a manner that they have never done before.

One of the most important things to remember is that you must create killer content each time you intend to create a post. Your content should be able to draw traffic to your blog – you must therefore write posts that get loads of comments, Facebook shares, pins and can get easily optimized for search engines.

In a nutshell, this would mean:

Amazing content = Killer blog post = Viral traffic = Great money

Reviewing some of the key action items from this chapter:

- Create a calendar of events and use it religiously
- Schedule a brainstorming session with yourself every week
- Write every single day – whether you like it or not, discipline is the key
- Create killer content that can get viral traffic

CHAPTER THREE: KEEPING IT CLEAN – PLAIN AND SIMPLE

Well, we live in a visual world and we like to see everything well organized. Here is the bitter truth – you can create an amazing calendar, write awesome content and maintain an incredible level of discipline. However, if the entire package does not sell….well, you are doomed.

Imagine a reader visiting your blog. Now, this is what they notice – there are five main colors, with some really pretty flowers in the background, colorful stripes in the header and a long footer that makes absolutely no sense. So, even though they are reading killer content, they are distracted by too much information available on your blog.

Your site may seem to be the most appealing site on earth to you, but it is definitely not pretty if your readers find it cluttered.

I would suggest a clean, simple, organized, easy to navigate design with fewer colors and more white space.

If you have been blogging for some time now, it is time to take a step back and reflect upon the following questions:

- Is your blog too cluttered or unorganized?
- Does your navigation make sense?
- Can your readers locate what they are looking for?
- Are your fonts easy to read?
- Can a newcomer visiting your blog get an idea (in thirty seconds) of what your blog is about and the kind of posts they can expect?
- Do all your posts have a clear call to action?
- Are your images high quality, appealing images?

The navigation toolbar in your blog should make things extremely easy for your readers. They must be able to find posts that they are looking for in just thirty seconds.

Take some time to create categories and then fit those categories into subtopics.

Categorize every post and eliminate categories that do not make sense. Highlight your best content in a manner that it stands out. How about including a 'most popular posts' section on your sidebar?

Wrap your content in a tasteful manner – a manner that people want to see. This means that your content must be presented in a neat and organized manner.

Here are some great and neat blog designs that I love:

As you notice the below designs, you will see that none of these blogs look alike. *The only common thing in these blogs is that they let their content show through*.

As you get to creating and maintaining your blog, you must understand the importance of images that you will use on your blog.

Here are some photography rules that you must stick to:

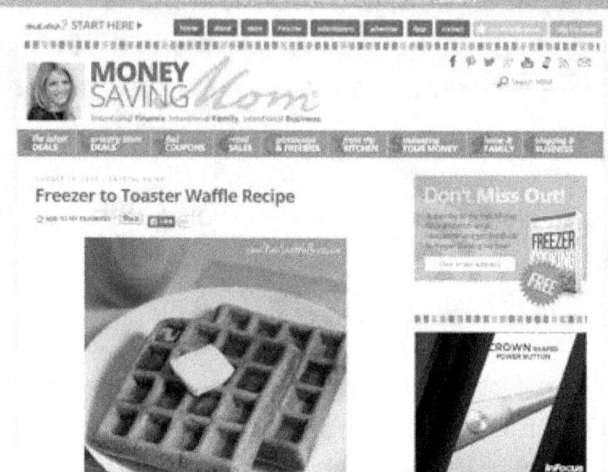

http://moneysavingmom.com/

http://www.ahaparenting.com/blog

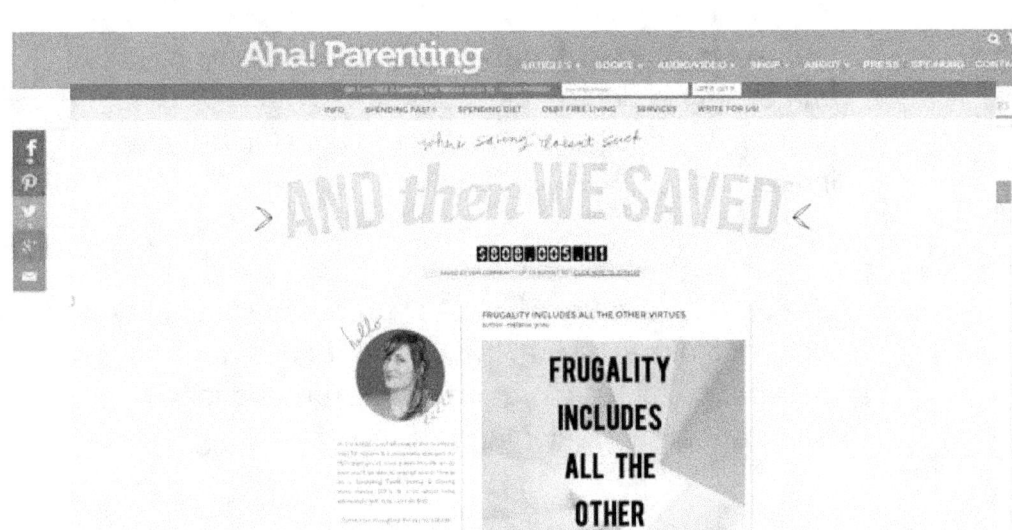

Invest in a good camera: Investing in a great camera is extremely important – your camera must be able to provide high quality images that your readers will drool over.

Be aware of the lightening: Good lightening is immensely important as you get ready to click a picture. Try and get most of your shoots in bright, indirect light.

Get a clean background: As you get ready to click a picture, make sure that the background is not distracting. A clean, organized background is important for a great image.

Try and make your images Pin-worthy. Remember, when used correctly, Pinterest is more powerful than Facebook, Google+ or Twitter.

Pin-worthy posts are always a combination of great content and captivating images.

Colorful images capture more attention than monochromatic ones. Warm colors are more likely to be re-pinned than cool colors. Close up shots and pins without faces stand a greater chance to be re-pinned.

Now, here is the thing – people collect and pin images they like – only because these images look super appealing to them. Converting your pins to page views implies that you have gone a step ahead and used Pinterest to the fullest.

Here are some examples of great images – the ones that are generally re-pinned and generate more traffic:

Source: www.pinterest.com

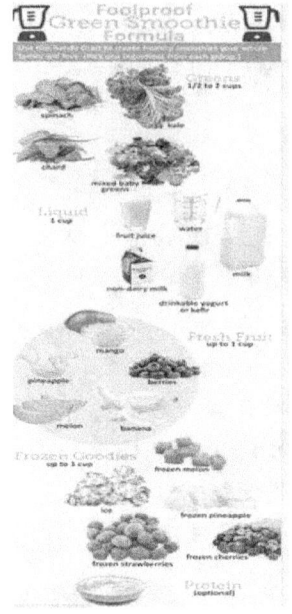

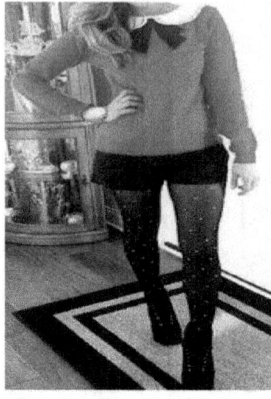

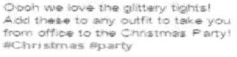

Oooh we love the glittery tights!
Add these to any outfit to take you
from office to the Christmas Party!
#Christmas #party

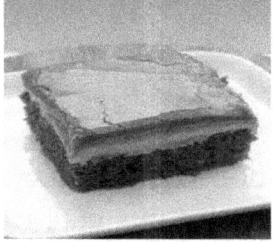

Peanut Butter Fudge cake- I Love
the combination of chocolate and
peanut butter!

And now, time for visiting the action items from this
chapter:

- You must revisit your blog design and develop a
  plan on the changes that you would like.
- Ensure that your design is simple and clean – free
  from unnecessary clutter.

- Create a well thought out navigation bar that tells your readers where to find stuff that they are looking for.
- Create pin-worthy blog posts - using content that rocks and high quality images that attract attention.

CHAPTER FOUR: BUILDING TRAFFIC

Before I begin talking about the limitless ways to build traffic to your blog, it is important to mention that you must not try to grow your platform if your blog is not ready yet.

Always remember that sustainable blog traffic growth can only happen if your content rocks. Having somebody visit your blog once is just one thing – but having them to come back again and again is another and that is the reason why awesome content is a necessity if you want to profit from your blog.

Here are some of the traditional ways to build traffic on your blog:

WORD OF MOUTH

Word of mouth is a great way to start building traffic on your blog – you tell your friends about your blog, who in turn tell their family and friends and that is how your list of readers increases – in case your content is read worthy.

Before you begin talking to people about your blog, spend some time crafting your elevator pitch. This is a thirty second overview of what your blog is about and how readers can benefit from it. Once you are ready with the pitch, practice it, hone it and own it.

Here are some ideas about how to build word of mouth publicity for your blog:

- How about sending a quick reminder to everyone in your address book whenever you publish a new blog post?
- Every time, you publish a new blog post, share it with a comment on your Facebook page and ask for feedback from relatives and friends.
- Have an inexpensive bumper sticker printed with your web address – this is how a number of people with get to know about your blog and begin reading it.
- Politely ask people you know and trust to spread the word around – you could ask them in person or include a link at the end of each blog post.

Remember, most first time bloggers feel embarrassed promoting their blog and asking for feedback. This is completely natural and should not discourage you from seeking support. Your friends may even mock at you initially. Once again, don't get discouraged by this and just continue promoting your blog. Think of it as your business and promote it as if you were promoting any other business.

COMMENTING ON OTHER BLOGS

You may have heard about shameless commenting on other, bigger blogs in order to drive traffic.

Well, here is the deal – while bloggers pretty much love to get comments, it is important to realize that they hate spammers – you just CANNOT scam the traffic these seasoned bloggers worked incredibly hard to build.

A better approach here is to read the blogs that you like – especially the ones that you feel have a great crossover traffic – and leave a thoughtful comment with your blog URL only if you genuinely have to say something. This means that your comments have to be genuine, straight from your heart. If your comments are genuine and insightful, they may lead other readers from the blog to reach out to you via your blog.

PROMOTE OTHER BLOGS

If you already have a sound database of readers, this 'pay it forward' approach can work wonders for your own blog.

Promoting another blogger can be as simple as linking back to another blogger whose post inspired any of your posts. Most blogs have trackbacks on their blog posts – this means that if you link a person's blog, they will automatically get a notification that you linked their blog. Now, I can't vouch for others, but whenever I receive such an alert, I definitely go and check the blog of the person who linked me. And that is human psychology – *most people do that, by default!*

Remember, the more you focus on building other people's blogs without accepting anything in return – the more it comes back to you in many different ways.

NETWORKING

Networking can open new doors for your blogging business. Apart from forging genuine friendships, you get the opportunity to grow your blog. I must mention here that 'true, genuine friendships' come first. If you make friends with the intention of growing your business, your friends can see right through your eyes.

The best way to connect with other bloggers is via blog conferences. This is a highly misunderstood profession and I can't tell you how amazing it is to be in the company of like-minded people who understand what you do for a living.

Here are few things that you can do at your first networking event:

Focus on making new connections: Even though you will be tempted to attend all sessions in order to make up for the money that you spent, don't fall into the trap and if possible, spend some time going out for coffee with the girl you met at breakfast or taking a small nap because you were busy chatting all night with your roommate, who is now your friend.

Find a roommate: Most blogging conferences have Facebook groups with a roommate connection thread – use that and get a roommate. Even if you and your roommate do not convert into overnight best friends, there is something really comforting about knowing at least one person in the group.

Listen more, speak less: The best way to learn is through listening – ask as many questions as you can and listen to the answers in the most genuine manner possible. There is a reason God gave us two ears and one mouth.

Listening and being genuinely interested in the conversation is a gift that you can give to other people at the conference and in the process, this can help you win genuine friends too. You will also be amazed at the amount of learning this can get you.

Engage in meaningful conversations: Imagine meeting a new person and just handing over your business card. What a turn off!

Focus on real conversations, not card swapping. I don't even keep the cards of people who I have not had a great conversation with. If you are genuinely interested in developing a relationship and don't know what to say, ask a question.

Don't let your new found friendship fade away: If you get a chance to develop authentic connections and are lucky enough to find somebody as amazing as you are, don't let the friendship fade away after the conference. Start reading their blogs, read their comments, send an occasional 'Hi', connect on Facebook – nurture the relationship.

GUEST POSTS

If done properly, guest posts have an amazing potential to drive traffic to your own blog. The key to a great guest post is to not post on a site with a similar audience but to write something so great that your host's readers are driven to your site in order to read more of what you write. If you are interested in guest posting on other sites, make sure that you ask for guidelines and always submit original content. Also, do not try to be overly familiar – since this is not 'your' audience. You are writing for somebody else's audience. Submit your best content and never make your post self-promotional.

BUILD YOUR E MAIL LIST

'Building an email list' model is extremely impactful when you want to reach out to an audience that can be converted into a sales funnel that you want to use in order to sell your expensive courses or physical products. This model is extremely effective for online marketers. However, for stay at home mommy's, this model may sometimes backfire – most of them will NEVER be interested in buying a $450 course.

Having said that, I still feel that building an email list is important. You can connect with your audience via newsletters and share news about your upcoming e-books and courses. I personally use Aweber to build my list, but I have also heard raving reviews about MailChimp.

As you build your email list, remember to place the subscribe button at a prominent place in your blog. Create some nice freebies for your subscribers – these could range from recipe books to goal setting and time management guides – just make sure that you are adding value to your readers.

Always promote the incentive that you offer on social media

UNDERSTAND SEARCH ENGINE OPTIMIZATION

As you create content, remember to create content that is SEO friendly. You must remember that Google's only goal is to display the best possible content for a particular search. The extremely sophisticated Google algorithms look at everything ranging from the content on the web page to the time visitors spent on the page. Another important thing to remember is that Google cannot be tricked via SEO. Here are some things that you must know in order to create a blog post that is Search Engine Optimized.

Title Tag: The title tag refers to words that show up at the very top of your browser window when you open a particular web page. The default title tag is generally the title of your post. However, it can be further optimized – remember that you can change the title tag and make it as long as you want, but Google will only read the first seventy characters. *You must therefore focus on optimizing the first seventy characters.*

Meta description: The default meta description is the first 150 words of your post. You can change it too – it helps in telling Google what your post is about.

Meta Keywords: Meta keywords are the search phrases that you like to see associated with your post.

They are more helpful in browsers such as Yahoo or Bing.

UNDERSTANDING THE POWER OF SOCIAL MEDIA

You may probably be familiar with the numerous options of social media – Facebook, Twitter, Pinterest, Instagram, Google+, StumbleUpon, LinkedIn, Snapchat, Reddit, etc.

Now, here is the point – I do not want you to use all the options listed here. In fact, most social media is a waste of time. Since you are treating your blog as your business, your time on social media must be measured in terms of ROI. You may have over a million Twitter followers. However, if none of them translate into readers….well, no point then!

You must work on developing your presence on platforms where your readers tend to be. As an example, for blogs targeted at women aged between 25-55, the ideal social media platform would be Facebook or Pinterest. For a blog that focuses on entrepreneurs or job seekers between the age group 25-40, the ideal social media platform would be LinkedIn.

Figure out where your audience is and use that platform – you want them to come back to your blog and read about what you have to offer.

As you focus on building your followers, remember *it is always quality that matters over quantity*. While it seems nice to have over one million followers (and I am sure a lot of them would be disengaged), it is nicer to have around 10,000 actively engaged followers.

As you build your Pinterest home page or your Facebook page, make sure that you use your blog name as your Pinterest and Facebook name. Be sure to include your blog address too.

Join as many collaborative boards as you can and be active – pin the relevant content on multiple boards. You could join the Pinterest Collaborative Boards group on Facebook.

And now, time for action plan from this chapter:

- Start talking about your blog with family and friends. Have some business cards printed and create an elevator pitch. Practice it at least once every day and OWN it.

- Read and comment on other people's blogs.
- Promote other bloggers by featuring their posts, or linking to a blog post that you really liked.
- Attend blog conferences, network with other bloggers and make friends.
- Create an incentive for people who subscribe to your e mail list (this could be anything from a free book or course to a physical item that they avail when they purchase something)
- Optimize your website and each blog post that you write, being careful not to spam your readers with a bunch of keywords.
- Do not focus on each and every social media platform available out there. Instead, focus on the platforms that can get you maximum readers.
- Determine your objectives before going for a paid Facebook promotion.
- Work on converting your new visitors into regular blog readers.

CHAPTER FIVE: HONEY, WHERE IS THE MONEY?

If you have managed to build a great blog with some awesome traffic, then the possibilities to monetize your blog can be limitless.

If you are really looking at building your blog for profit, then it is important to understand that rushing things up might not help. Almost all full time bloggers (who use their blog to earn a living), have been regularly blogging for at least three years now. It takes time to build steady traffic that can help you earn a living. You may choose to run advertisements, use affiliate links or work with brands from day one, but you must remember that the traffic that you get on your blog will ultimately determine your ability to monetize your blog.

Therefore, the first thing that you must concentrate on is to 'Go Slow.' Stay away from the quick fix money making hacks and focus on the big picture. Look at how you can create awesome content and ensure that you are building your base of readers. Do not agree to write sponsored posts or host giveaways for products that you are not even convinced about but can get you some quick bucks. Instead, focus on writing content that gets more readers.

Substantial research has been conducted to prove that there is a definite relationship between the number of monthly page views a blog gets and the amount of money the blog owner earns.

Let us look at some of the methods that can help you in monetizing your blog (once you have enough readers):

Ad Networks: Advertising networks such as Google AdSense, Media.net , PulsePoint.com , BlogHer, etc. work with a large number of advertisers who pay the network to place their ad on your site. Depending on the ad network, you could receive a cost per thousand views or a pay per click payment. Sometimes, it is a combination of these two things.

Once your advertisements are in place, you do not have to do anything. You make money by simply sitting there. The only flipside to this is the inconsistent ad traffic. If you happen to be at the right place at the right time, you may earn a lot of money for a while. However, as trends begin to fall, your income may begin to fluctuate.

This implies that revenue from ad networks is incredible when you can capture it. It also implies that you need to exercise caution as you rely on revenue from advertisements. You must diversify your income.

Therefore, if you want to earn profit from your blog, you can let the ad network be your important revenue stream, but you can never let it be your only revenue stream.

The highest paying ad network is Google AdSense.

BlogAds allows bloggers to sell their ad space, set their own prices, and even reject or accept ads.

As you begin using these ad networks, you must learn to optimize the placement of these advertisements – so that you get maximum clicks and revenue. Research proves that the best placement is directly above, below, or to the left of your primary blog content. Make sure to use a darker color for ad placements.

You can also use content based advertising. Remember, users who visit your blog for its content are more likely to click on the relevant products that you advertise on your blog.

Private advertising: Private advertising is any paid advertisement or link on your site that is paid directly by the company that is advertising, rather than a network. It is generally a specific ad at a specific spot that stays up for a limited period of time.

In order to work with brands directly, you must clearly define your brand strategy and figure out nice, innovative ways through which you could offer private advertising on your website in the most authentic manner possible.

You must be able to determine how you want to work with brands. In order to sell your site to various brands, spend some time packaging your blog. Create an attractive advertising booklet that provides the brands you intend to work with, with a description of your blog along with the traffic statistics and opportunities available. You may want to consider setting up a specific email address solely for the purpose of advertising requests.

Affiliate advertising: Affiliate advertising is an ad or a link to a product or a company that results in a commission only if the click on that ad leads to a sale. This could include Amazon links or links through other websites such as Pepperjam Network , ShareASale, E Junkie, etc.

The most successful affiliate sales are a result of creating a relationship of trust with your readers. Your readers will buy the things that you recommend because they trust you – they trust what you write and are happy with the manner in which you keep them engaged.

The payout for Amazon sales is fairly low (around 5%) in comparison to other affiliate programs. However, the best thing about Amazon is their user friendly interface which allows you to link to link to any of their pages or products. Now, imagine somebody clicking on the affiliate link, reaching the Amazon site, and in the process of surfing for a $5 book, buying a $500 coffee machine!

Yes…this is also possible with Amazon – they sell everything under the sun and the person who bought the coffee machine used your affiliate link, which means you get a commission on that. *Cool, isn't it?*

The only way to increase your affiliate sales is by producing awesome content and paying attention to the kind of things that your readers are using and buying. Be honest with your readers and share links for things that you actually use or places that you actually visit. Always ensure that your links are relevant.

Sponsored posts and Brand promotion: Another popular monetization strategy is to work directly with brands to promote their products within a post or series of posts. These can be posts that are written on a topic provided by the sponsor, product reviews, or paid product giveaways.

Selling products: You could use your blog to sell your e-books, your e-courses or even items such as t-shirts, tote bags, handmade decorative items, etc. And the results are self-explanatory – you get to market your products via your blog, and you also get to earn awesome profits – with practically zero investment.

Selling services: Depending on the niche that you are comfortable with, you could sell services such as local classes, hobby ideas or even online consulting services such as virtual feng shui and vaastu consultation.

<u>Writing and Speaking opportunities</u>: Many popular speakers get their first speaking assignment through writing a successful blog post. You never know, you may be the next one in the line!

Let us look at some of the action items from this chapter:

- You must take it slow – realize the every blogger earns income differently and almost nobody earns it overnight.
- Figure out what resources you would like to use and decide accordingly. You do not have to use all monetization channels. Identify the voice of your blog and see what fits best.
- Be authentic with your readers – do not advertise products that you do not believe in or would not use personally.

CHAPTER SIX: STAYING ORGANIZED AND AIMING FOR THE PERFECT WORK LIFE INTEGRATION

Well, blogging seems to be an incredibly easy profession. You can be sitting in your PJs, sipping your cup of coffee, watching over your adorable kids and still be working.

The best piece of advice that I have ever received when it comes to blogging is to work smarter. There are only 24 hours in a day and when you are blogging for profit, there is always so much that can still be done.

We live in an extremely connected world, so the process of liking a friend's blog, or commenting on somebody's blog or even responding to a comment that you just received on your blog, can become a 24/7 activity.

Think about your blog as your business and set your own boundaries. Create work timings and be strict with yourself.

Create a to-do list and ensure that you follow your daily calendar or events.

Do not procrastinate and get the big things accomplished first.

Take regular breaks and delete what is not essential (or not important) in the important/ urgent matrix.

Aim at bringing your inbox to zero every single day.

And most important, *give yourself permission to enjoy life – to get out of your home office and have some fun. You do not have to get everything done. And you must be prepared for that.*

*Bonus Book 2

Blogging for Beginners

A Beginners Guide to Blogging about Your Passion

Chapter 1: What is Blogging About?

Blogging is about writing information and getting paid for it. If you've never done it before you probably don't really get what that means but it's simple enough to understand. When you 'blog' about something it means you're creating articles and almost diary-like entries that usually about a certain topic. This isn't always true, some people will blog about a variety of subject, but most will stick with one thing they know a lot about. You also will want to make sure that you're focusing on something you enjoy because if you're trying to make money you want to stick with that topic.

You are able to create your own website entirely for your blog or you can create a webpage on another website. If you really want to make the most money from blogging you'll want to get a website with a decent host. There are several hosting companies that will provide you with a website of your own but keep in mind that the better companies are going to charge you some money. You do have the ability to start with a cheaper blog and then transfer it to another host, however this is going to take more time and be more difficult. It may also be more confusing for your readers if you already have a fan base when you switch the information over.

Now we're getting a little ahead of ourselves so let's back up a bit. A blog can be about absolutely anything you want. If you enjoy writing then you can write a blog about how to write. If you like dogs you can blog about that. Choose something that you are highly knowledgeable about and that you can provide information for others about. You want to have something to offer anyone who comes to read your blog after all. If you don't they aren't likely to continue reading your blog.

Once you've created the topic that you want to use it's time to start blogging. What you do in a blog is create articles that are based on the specific topic that you've chosen. You want to focus on things that are going to get your readers interested in your topic. Talk to them about your experiences, your knowledge or even teach them courses. You'll be able to explain a lot of information to them and you may actually be surprised how much of a response you get. Plus you get to have fun.

Typically those who are blogging will also keep track of their blogs so that they can write several times a month or even several times a week. Generally the more blog posts you write the better your readership is going to be. That's because your readers want to learn more and they are going to show up whenever they can count on new information (so try to keep it regular). If they know you aren't going to post frequently or they can't count on when you're going to post you'll find yourself losing viewers.

Chapter 2: Starting the Blog

If you want to start a blog you need to come up with your topic first. Think about all the things you know and really like. This is your basis for creating a blog. Once you've come up with a few ideas start thinking of some sample titles. Once you get more advanced you may be able to start multiple blogs but when you're just beginning you want to make sure you focus all your attention on one blog. Anymore and you might get distracted, confused or even struggle to keep up the information you need for your readers.

Look over the list of potential topics that you have and try to figure out which is going to be the best. You want to pick something that's going to give you plenty of opportunity to write more titles and you also want to make sure that you have a good basis to start with. From there you'll be able to develop what your basis is going to be and you'll be able to better understand what your reader base is going to be.

Once you've created the topic you need to find the host that you want to use. Make sure that you choose something that is going to give you a lot of benefits but isn't going to give you too many ads (which can detract from your reader base). This is not going to be cheap but it doesn't have to be extremely expensive either. Be willing to compromise a little bit. You need to invest in yourself to really start off your blog.

Next, make sure you spend some time creating your website. You want to make it look interesting and user-friendly.

Make sure that you have headings for different pages and that they make sense. Be sure that your entire website has a cohesive look. You don't want it to look cheap or to look bland and boring. These things are going to lose you a lot of readers and they are definitely going to hurt your ability to make a profit as well (once you get there).

The best thing you can do is look at other websites in the same genre. Look at what other people are posting and how they've set up your website. That's how you're going to understand what your readers are really looking for. It's also going to help you make your website look like it belongs in the genre.

Create your first blog post as more of an introduction to yourself and your blog in general. You don't want to just jump into a lot of information because you'll confuse your readers who won't know why they should trust you or what right you have to tell them anything about the topic. So instead, you want to create an initial blog post that is going to introduce you and explain how and why you are the person that they should trust to learn more about your topic. Use it as an opportunity and then make sure that this post is there for anyone that may show up later on to read your blog, after you've established yourself. It may turn into your 'about me' page, for example.

The post should explain all of your qualifications such as education or work experience. It should also explain how you gain your information, whether this is a hobby or firsthand knowledge in some other way. Then explain why you are interested in the subject and give a brief overview of just a few of the things that you have knowledge about. This is going to help you gain additional readers because they are going to believe that you have the type of information they are looking for. This makes them more inclined to come back and check for new posts frequently. You may even want to follow up this introduction post with your first post about your topic.

Make sure that your first real information post is giving some information that is interesting or unknown. The more interesting the information that you give the more you're going to get repeat readers. That's because they realize that the information you have is actually going to be valuable. Even if they already know what you've talked about they will realize that not everyone does and this makes them believe that you really are the expert that you claim to be. You also get more attention from beginners in the field because they realize your information is pretty great as well. Having more readers is going to translate into getting you even more money, but only if you're careful and follow along with some of the other information we're going to talk about later.

Chapter 3: Making Money With Your Blog

So we've talked about what a blog is and what you need to do in order to start your blog. So far we've only talked about how you're going to spend money however, and not how you're going to make money. Well it's actually fairly simple to start making money with your blog. You just need to take a little bit of extra time and you need to make sure that you are providing some high quality information. You can make a small amount of money in one simple way, ads.

Ads will allow you to make money because they are simply posted onto your website without you needing to do anything. If you work with a program such as Google AdSense you will be able to get ads that relate to your particular blog. You can also get sponsored ads from different companies that produce products that are related to your blog or even that you personally recommend in that area. This is going to help you get revenue because the company will give you a small amount of money just for letting them post an ad.

If you want to make even more money then you want to make sure that you are getting involved in more than just a posting fee. You want to get a pay-per-click program as well. In this program you will get a set fee just to let the ad post to your website. You will also get a little bit extra every time someone clicks on the ad on your site. This is a way to upgrade the amount of money that you make but it's actually only the midrange. If you really want to make more money you can work on a partnership program. This will allow you to get some money from the people who post ads on your website if someone clicks through your website and purchases something. You can often get a share of the profits that the company makes.

Keep building up your blog and your following and you'll be able to get even more benefits and more revenue. That's because the more people you have following you the more your page is worth. That means you can sell that space for ads to someone that's willing to pay a lot more. There are a few important things to keep in mind at this point however.

The first thing to understand is that your readers want to find out more information that they can trust. That means they don't want to go to your page and realize that you're trying to convince them to buy something that isn't any good. If you start recommending products that they can't trust then they will stop trusting you and that means they will stop coming to your blog. Unfortunately, too many ads (something that will get you more revenue) is also going to turn away readers. If they have to spend too much time sorting through ads to get to the content they are going to find a different web page that can give them at least close to the information without all those ads.

Make sure that you are consistently posting new information. If something new happens in your field you want to talk about it. People are relying on you to give them information in that area after all and if they can't find the latest and most relevant information with you then they are going to go somewhere else. Another thing is to make sure that you are posting often. You need to post at least once per week if you are hoping to make any kind of money with your blog. If you post less frequently then your readers aren't going to believe you have the information they need.

The problem with posting frequently is that it's easy to run out of topics and things to talk about. Don't let this happen to you. Make sure that you are constantly searching for more information on your topic and that you're writing about everything you learn. If you learn something new during your research don't be afraid to let your readers know about it. Don't be afraid to let them know that you didn't know this before either. It's going to make you seem human and that makes you more relatable and more interesting to your reader.

Finally, when all else fails, ask the question 'what do you want to know about this topic.' Ask all of your readers on an open forum, through an email or in a survey. This will give you the ability to talk about the topics that are interesting to your readers and that's going to make them stay even more because they will know that you listened to them and you find them important.

Chapter 4: Advanced Money Making Opportunities

Using ads and companies to create revenue for yourself is definitely a great way to make money. It's a great way to get started. But if you really want to start making the big money then there's even more you need to do. If you want to quit your current day job you need to spend your time and effort on these larger methods of making money because they're actually going to make that money much faster than anything else you do.

You can start charging for your blog. Look at what you've built. Look at how much you've been able to gain and how much viewership you've gained. This is going to be important because it shows that you have something other people want. What you want to do is start charging people to read your blog. You don't have to charge for all the content; you may decide to keep a good amount of it free to anyone that cares to read it. On the other hand, you'll want to create some premium content that depends on a fee rather than just giving it away.

Remember, you've established yourself as an expert in your field now. You've created a way of drawing in new readers and you deserve to make the most out of your blog. So do it. Start charging either by the article or for a monthly subscription to your premium articles and then make sure that they are worth it. You'll need to spend a little bit more time on those articles, making sure they are higher quality and making sure also that they are going to improve the lives of those that are reading them. Your regular readers will probably check out the premium subscription first (in fact you may want to give them a free preview to help sell them on the idea of purchasing the subscription and letting others know about it too).

The next thing is to stop selling your ad space. Stop letting other people post information on your blog. Don't sell their products for them. Don't recommend that people buy them. You're going to completely wipe out advertising from your blog. Now you may be thinking this is madness. You're probably looking at the money you're already making and thinking, but I'm going to lose all of my income if I turn away all of my investors. The truth is that you will for a short while, but you're going to make it back and then some.

As you started developing your blog you created yourself as someone that can be trusted. You showed your readers that you had plenty of knowledge in your field and that they could rely on you to always give them the truth. They found out that you wouldn't recommend products that weren't any good and that you really knew what you were talking about. This was what you really wanted and it's the reason you really wanted to post information about other products at the beginning of your journey.

Now that you've fully established yourself it's time to start creating your own products. Look at your blog. Look at what you've been writing about. Have you ever thought that you could create a better dog toy? Or that you could create a better journal? Or that you could teach people how to start their own business better than anyone else? If you have then you're already one step ahead of the game. If you haven't ...

well it's about time you started thinking that way because chances are you probably can.

The best thing you can do to make some money for yourself is start creating your own products that are also in your field. Consider what you know about the field and then spend a little time and money developing products that will make the lives of your readers even better. Now I understand that we just told you to spend some money. You'll need to spend some money in order to develop the products but just think of how much money you'll be able to make when you actually start to sell those products.

The important thing is that you have a good following and a following that trusts you before you start investing in your own products. If you don't you could end up spending a lot of money and not actually get anything out of it. Once you've developed all of these things you're going to need to reach out to someone that can create the products that you need. You don't need to spend time actually developing and creating them for yourself. Instead, just take some time finding the right person to do so for you.

Now, once you have the product you need to make sure that you market it. You may want to start with only a couple products but don't be afraid to branch out and create a range of different products for yourself. You'll be able to get a lot more people interested in your products because they already trust you with everything else that you're saying. The more products you have and the more you tell people about them the better off you will be.

What you need to consider is striking a balance. You need to promote your products and let everyone know about them. At the same time however, you want to make sure that you are not turning your entire blog into a scam to try and sell your products. This will turn away a lot of your readers and you'll lose out on sales as well as losing out on the readers who can bring others to your website. The better your products are the more you'll be able to sell and the more word is going to start getting out about them.

The next thing you can work on selling is courses. Try to help your readers in as many ways as necessary. Create videos that will show them how to do certain things or how to use different skills. Some of these videos may be completely free. Others you may want to charge for. The key is deciding which content is worth the most money and pricing it accordingly. Don't be afraid to charge more money for better, more important or longer content. Each of these things is going to improve your revenue and it's going to make sense to those who are checking your blog as well because they realize that they pay more for the information that is going to be the most valuable.

Outside of generic videos you can also create a webinar which will allow your readers to see more information and go through an entire course designed to teach them a brand new skill. Once they've completed the webinar they will be able to do more for themselves and this is very important to just about anyone. Make sure you take your time to create quality webinars. Nothing is going to annoy your readers more than spending money on something that isn't valuable to them. If you create quality content and teach them something they need to know it's going to keep them coming back.

Chapter 5: Keep it Going (Conclusion)

At this point you will be making some good money on your blog. You're probably going to be ready to quit your day job and well you should be (if you haven't done it already). You want to make sure that you keep everything going the way you have previously but you also need to know some important tips to keep in mind throughout the entire process. They are going to make it easier to attract new readers and definitely much easier to keep those readers coming back.

The first thing you need to know about is content. We talked about keeping your content high quality but this is even more important when you're just starting out and once you start charging for articles. You need to make sure that the articles your readers are finding are going to help them in some way. This could be teaching them a new skill or helping them with a difficult problem. What you may not know is that you don't need to actually write the content for yourself.

If you are interested in building a blog but don't have the writing skills then you can actually hire someone to create the blog for you. They will take the time out of their day to write the individual articles, add images and maybe even post them to the website for you. You pay them for these services and then you collect a larger fee from the blog itself through revenue. Of course, there are plenty of sites that you can choose from where you can find a blog writer and a website manager. Just make sure you're finding someone who can create quality content. You don't want your quality to suffer and lose you readers.

Another thing you should know is SEO. This stands for Search Engine Optimization and it relates to the way that other people are able to find your blog. Within every single industry there are several key words and phrases that people search for the most often when they use a search engine (such as Google or Yahoo). These phrases are the ones that you want to make sure that you use in your articles and throughout your website. The more you use them the better your rankings are going to be on these search engines, at least, to a point.

The important thing is to use these key words and phrases when they make sense. For example, let's say the keyword that I'm trying to use is book bag. 'My book bag is much stronger than the book bag that is currently sitting next to your book bag on the pile of book bags.' Does this sound natural to you? Did it tell you anything about why my book bag is stronger than yours? No and no. You don't want to do this in your article because search engine algorithms, the thing that figures out where in the search engine ranking your website should go, is as smart as the average person in most ways. That means it will find this sentence, rank the use of key words high and rank the worth of those key words low. Your webpage will sink to the bottom of the list.

The information that you post needs to contain key words but it also needs to be useful. By balancing out these two important aspects you're going to get more readers because when they search for key words your website is going to pop up. If the article that they find is useful compared to the information that they are looking for they are more likely to check out a few more of your articles. If the information isn't useful, like my little book bag post above, they are going to leave your webpage and keep looking for something different. This is not good for you because chances are if they look for something else in the future they will scroll right past your listing because of their past experiences.

By using only quality content, high SEO content and someone else to create your blog posts you will be able to make more money and actually spend less time on your blog. It's a win-win and the complete opposite of what we told you was going to happen earlier on. That's because, once you're established, you don't have to put as much work or effort into getting what you need out of your website.

*Bonus Book 3

How To Raise Your Credit Score

The Ultimate Guide To Your Total Money Makeover: Tips and Strategies- For Saving Money, Credit Repair, and Becoming Debt Free

Introduction

Hello, I want to thank you and congratulate you for taking the time to read, *The Ultimate Guide to Your Total Money Makeover: Tips and Strategies-For Saving Money, Credit Repair, and Becoming Debt Free*.

This book contains proven steps and strategies on how to save money and get yourself in better financial shape.

In this book we're going to talk about three different aspects of financial success. We're going to explain how you can and should go about saving more money and what you need to do in order to make sure that you eliminate debt.

Getting yourself in the best possible financial shape is important to your overall success in life. After all, without the right amount of money to support yourself and your family it's nearly impossible to do everything that you want and that's what life is all about right? You want to be able to enjoy yourself as much as possible.

But in order to truly live a happy life you need to make sure that you are financially stable and that means saving money, getting your credit in good shape and eliminating debt.

Thanks again for downloading this book, I hope you enjoy it!

Chapter 1: Budgeting Your Money, The Easy Way

If you're looking to get out of debt the most important thing you need to do is make sure you know where your money is going. You want to make sure that you understand how much you owe to each place, company or person and then you'll be able to take the time and make the effort to actually create a budget that works.

For many people, the very idea of creating a budget is daunting. How can you possibly figure out how much money you should send to everyone when you don't even really know how much money you have or how much money you owe or which one you should pay off first? There's just too many questions involved and you find yourself completely thrown off and confused.

That's why step one is making sure you know how much you owe and to whom. Start by making a list of all the information you have. List the amount of money that's owed, who you owe it to and whether the amount is currently a collection or is just 'past due.' Both of these categories are important but knowing the difference will help you understand which to pay off first.

Past due accounts are those that you owe to a credit company but they are still contacting you asking for payment. They haven't revoked your credit yet, they're just tacking on a lot of fines, fees and interest for as long as you don't pay the account. These accounts are going to look back on your credit report (which we'll talk about later) but they aren't going to be as bad as collection accounts. These types of accounts are generally capable of being paid off in monthly payments (regular credit card payments)

A collection account is one where the credit company has completely given up on getting their money back. What they do is they sell the debt to a collection agencies and that agency attempts to get the money back from you. This is money that has been overdue for a long period of time and you know owe the entire amount is due all at the same time. In some instances you can get the company to take payments or accept a lower settlement but you're generally responsible for the entire account.

When you're working on creating a budget you want to make sure you're paying at least a little bit of money on each of your past due accounts because this encourages them to keep the account open. They want to get as much money from you as possible and if they choose to close the account and turn it into a collection that won't happen. So they keep the account open as long as you continue to pay (even if you aren't making full monthly payments and the fees are still racking up.

With a collection you need to contact the company if you want to attempt to make payments (usually not easy) or you need to pay off the entire amount (or settlement amount) all at the same time. This means you need to come up with all the money or you really can't do anything about the account.

When you create your budget you want to think about everything that you have coming into the home and then think about every bill that you have. The bills that are considered current you want to keep current. These are helping your credit score even as other past due bills are hurting it. These are bills like your lights, electricity, water and food. Make sure you have enough money set aside monthly to pay for all of these things. Determine how much money you need in order to pay off those current bills and then look at what's left over. A portion of this should go into a savings account. Try to get at least $50 to go to savings every month. This will help you slowly build up a little nest egg in case of emergencies.

The money that's left over needs to be divided over the rest of your past due bills. Try to at least reach the minimum payment amount on your credit cards or accounts that are considered past due. This will help you keep from getting additional fees for not meeting the minimum payment amount. If you can afford to pay the amount that's past due you'll be even better off but try to keep the account open. That means you want to keep some type of charge on the account so they don't close it.

If you're past due on an account it's more likely that they will close the account once they get your money. As we'll talk about in a later chapter, this isn't something that you want to happen. That means you want to keep a balance on the card but try to keep it current instead of past due. This will help you build your credit back up.

Once you've taken the minimum payment amount for each of your past due accounts try to see what's left. If there's anything left see if it will come close to the payoff amount for one of your collection accounts. If it's close you may be able to negotiate with the company (which we'll discuss in our chapter about collection agencies).

Your budget should go somewhere that you can see it easily and often. You don't want to mess up your budget because that's going to keep you on track with your spending and with paying off bills. That will get you out of debt faster and help you get back to having fun with your money (instead of giving it to everyone else for nothing).

Chapter 2: Dispute the Charges

You should always keep an eye on your credit report. There are plenty of credit card companies and even websites that will provide it to you completely free so make sure you're taking advantage of that feature. You'll be able to monitor if someone ever steals your identity and you're also going to be able to keep track of the accounts that are affecting your credit score both in positive and negative ways.

If you look at your credit report and see a lot of negative accounts, such as past due or collection accounts, consider whether they are accurate. Did you know that the credit reporting agencies are required by law to ensure that your credit report is 100% accurate at all times? If it's not they are required (also by law) to remove the incorrect information.

What this means to you is that, if the negative accounts on your credit report are not 100% accurate you can request to have them removed. What you want to do is review your report and consider which accounts may not be correct. Now keep in mind you're not allowed to dispute anything that is true. So if the negative account on your credit report is accurate you're supposed to leave it alone. If it's not, write a letter to the credit reporting agency (that's Transunion, Equifax or Experian) and ask them to remove it. Let them know why it needs to be removed and make sure you include your name, birthdate and social security number in the letter.

If you do this then the credit reporting agency is required to investigate and make sure the account is accurate. If it is then they will send you a letter verifying the account and request that if you have evidence that it's not accurate you send that information to them. If it is not accurate they must remove it from your credit report and your credit score will be updated to reflect it.

Writing letters to the credit reporting agencies doesn't always work 100%. Sometimes they will continue to tell you an account has been verified when you know it isn't accurate. If this happens you'll have to go above their heads and write to the original creditor, letting them know that the account is inaccurate and providing information that verifies this. This could be statements showing your bills were paid on time or letters indicating that they removed the account. Remember to send copies of these documents and not the actual letter.

Disputing false information can get a lot of accounts dropped and it can remove some of your debt because you won't have to pay for those collections or past due charges if you can prove that they are not accurate. Plus this is going to improve your credit score and repair your credit because the negative accounts are being removed.

Chapter 3: Negotiate With Credit Companies

Another thing not a lot of people know is that you can negotiate with credit companies. So you're able to take the collection letter they send you or a past due notice that has been sent to you and discuss it with them. In many cases they will take a lower amount than what's on the bill just so that they can guarantee they'll get something

Let's say you owe Discover $1,000. They really want to get their money so they send you a past due notice. But for several months you've ignored that past due notice and now they've sent it to collections. The collections agency may offer you a settlement. Maybe they say they'll take $900 if you just pay it to them right then and there. You have the opportunity to call them and request that they take a lesser amount.

If you talk to the collection agency and they agree to take a lesser amount you will have to send that payment in full. Make sure that when you send them the check you write out the words 'paid in full' on the check. Make a copy of the check for your own records as well. Once they cash that check your account is legally considered to be paid in full and they are no longer able to come after you for more money.

In many cases an original creditor or a collection agency will accept less than the bill is for just because they want to get something. They know that if you've ignored them for this long you may continue to do so and they may never be able to get any money out of you. In fact, a large number of people who have immense debts and a lot of collections out for them will just go bankrupt and then those companies never get anything. That's why they are willing to accept lower payments. A lower payment will guarantee them something for their trouble and it will allow them to close out the account.

Chapter 4: Cut the Credit Cards

If you're looking to save some money then you need to make sure you're spending less. That means getting rid of all those credit cards. If you have a lot of credit cards you're going to be tempted to use them and that's not going to help you save anything. So what you want to do is get rid of the credit cards.

One thing it's important to remember is that actually closing out your credit cards is probably going to decrease your credit score. When you have less available credit (the amount of money that the credit card companies allow you to spend) your amount of credit used increases. What you want to do is make sure that you keep a few credit cards so you have a decent amount of available credit. You want to avoid using them however.

If you're able to avoid the temptation to purchase things you can put one credit card in the back of your purse or wallet. Choose a card that will work anywhere such as a major credit card company. This is for emergencies only. An emergency doesn't mean you found something that you really want to have. It means that your car broke down and needs to be towed, or you run out of gas.

The rest of the credit cards you decide to keep should be locked up somewhere in your home. Put them in a safe or lockbox. This way you have to actively think about getting the card out again before you're able to actually use it. This will keep you from using the card in a spur of the moment fashion and will ensure that you still have it available if absolutely necessary.

Stop using credit cards as much as possible. This will allow you to save more money because you won't have to spend a lot of your money on credit card bills at the end of the month. Instead, you'll have all the money you would have spent on those bills left over to put in a savings account. Remember that budget you made at the beginning of this book and make sure that you stick to it. Don't spend too much of your money on things you don't need throughout the month.

Keep in mind that if you don't use your credit card at all it's eventually going to be taken away from you. That's because the credit card companies don't want to allow credit to someone that isn't going to do anything with it and eventually they will cancel your account. This is going to lower the amount of available credit you have and it's going to decrease your credit score.

The best thing to do is make one to two small purchases on your credit card every few months. Try to space out using different cards so that none of them get taken but you don't owe very much money each month. You want to keep the amount negligible. That means it's low enough that it really doesn't affect your overall budget. This is going to let you keep the card but, at the same time, it's not going to completely break the bank.

Chapter 5: Understanding Your Credit Report

Your credit report is not all that easy to understand. There are a lot of different categories in the report and that means you need to weigh out different things in order to make sure that your credit score is going to be high enough for you to get the things you want.

The best scores are those that are over 900 but not many people are actually able to achieve that. If your score is over a 700 you actually have really good credit and you're pretty much guaranteed any type of credit that you might apply for. But you want to keep in mind that different types of credit card companies or credit agencies will want a different score.

If your score is in the 600's you have a decent chance of getting credit in most places but not all. This isn't guaranteed however. There are plenty of agencies that will consider you a little bit of a risk.

Your credit score is actually an indication of how much of a risk it is to give you credit. When you first start out getting credit you have a low credit score. This tells the person checking your score that there is a high level of risk involved. They don't know if you're going to pay the bills or if you're going to rack up high amounts of charges. That's why your score is low. As you get more recorded payments your score will go up because the risk of you not paying for things is getting lower.

Now it's not just late payments or missed payments that are going to count against you in regards to your credit score. There are actually a lot of different factors that cause problems with your credit score (or improve your credit score)

So let's break them down a little and look at what's on your credit report.

Public records are one of the first things that show up on your credit report. These are the worst things you can have, judgments and tax liens against you. Any of these are going to make a big dent in your credit score and they're going to continue to work against you for a very long time (up to 7 years). You definitely don't want these if you can help it.

The next thing is going to be your credit items. These are credit cards, loans, mortgages and any other credit account that you've had in the past. Most accounts that are considered old (closed more than 10 years ago) will not report unless you've had a collection filed for that account.

Each of your credit items is going to count towards your credit score. Every on time payment is going to count in your favor and every late payment, missed payment or collection is going to count against you. Each balance is going to be reported as well and high balances are also going to count against you.

Remember we said before that you want to have a high available credit balance but you also want to have a low balance on the credit you're using. What the credit reporting agency does is look at how much you're able to spend on all of your credit cards and add that together. That's your available credit balance. They then look at how much money you owe on each of those cards and add that all together.

The amount owed is divided by the amount available and that's your total balance percentage. You want to keep this percentage low because that reflects well on your credit card. A high percentage is going to look bad and lower your credit score.

The total amount of accounts that you have as well as the types of accounts is going to count towards your score as well. You actually want to have a moderate number of accounts (more than 10) as long as you can keep them all current. You also want to have an assortment of accounts (credit cards, mortgages, car loans, student loans, etc.) this is going to improve your score as well.

Finally, the number of inquiries that you have will affect your score. You want to cut down on the amount of inquiries that you have because every one is a slight ding to your account. What these are is every time that you apply for credit. If you apply they check your credit score and when they check your credit score it goes down a little bit. These inquiries stay on your credit report for some time as well.

That's why you want to apply for credit infrequently and only if you're sure you're going to get it. Getting the credit will help improve your score more than it's going to hurt for the inquiry.

So all in all you want to make sure of a few important things in regards to your credit report:

- Have several different accounts (10 or more)

- Keep all accounts current

- Avoid public records

- Have a variety of types of accounts (loans and credit cards)

- Keep your available balance high

- Keep the balance in use low

- Don't apply for credit unless necessary

- Never apply for credit unless you're sure you'll be approved

- Dispute accounts that aren't correct

- Make payments on any past due accounts and pay off collections

By doing all of these things your credit score will actually increase over time. It will take some time and you're definitely going to need to work at it but you'll be able to bring your credit score back up. Once you're able to bring your score back up you'll find it even easier to get out of debt and you'll start saving better as well.

The reason your credit score is going to affect this is because your credit score actually has a lot to do with you getting approved for everything from credit cards to car loans to housing. It also has to do with the interest rates that you're given. As your score goes up you'll be able to request lower interest rates and that makes it even easier to pay off debts and stay out of debt in the long run. Staying out of debt means you have more money to put away towards your savings. So it's really a win all the way around.

Chapter 6: Ways You Never Knew You Could Raise Your Score

You can actually ask credit card companies to get rid of problems on your credit report even if you are actually in the wrong. What you want to do is simply call or write to the credit card company directly. Let them know that you understand you were late on a payment but point out your history and show that you have not been late in the past and you made a one-time mistake. (If you have been late frequently they probably won't work with you as much.).

Now if you have never made this mistake before or if you have rarely done it the credit card company may be willing to wave a late payment. This would mean that they take the late payment remark from your history and you may not even have to pay a fine. But by taking off the mark on your history they are improving your credit score. That one little late payment can be a big problem and it can result in your score taking a big hit. If it gets removed you no longer have to worry about it and your credit score could go up quite a bit.

Keeping old accounts open is another important way that you can improve your credit score. The oldest accounts that you have are actually improving your credit, whether they are positive or negative. What this means is you could have a long history of late payments with your oldest account but you're getting more positive marks on your credit from that account being so old than you are negative marks for the late payments. You don't ever want to close your oldest account unless you have no way around it. This account is doing great things for you.

Now if you have multiple accounts that are very close to the same age and one has a lot of negative marks you can close it. What you don't want to do is close the only account you have that's older than two years. (Of course, the older the account is the better it is for you.) Only close this account if there's an important reason for it or if you have another account that is very close to the same age and is giving you the same benefits when it comes to account history.

All those 'free quote' websites are actually hurting your credit score as well. You need to make sure that you are not signing up for a lot of those quotes. Even when you're searching for something like car insurance or health insurance you need to be careful. Free quotes may sound great but how do you think they're able to give you that quote? They need to know a little more about you in order to give you something that they can guarantee and that means they run your credit history and check out your credit score. That helps them to know whether you'll pay your bills or not and that affects your quote.

Pay your balance more than once a month. A lot of people use their credit cards for everything. That's either because it's easier to use instead of having to carry around a lot of cash, or because you just want to keep raking in rewards points that you can use for other things. Those are perfectly good reasons and if you're paying off the card every month you're not getting late charges or anything like that which is a benefit to you. On the other hand, you could be hurting your credit utilization rate.

Now you may be thinking, I pay it off every month so how could I be hurting my credit score? Well, when your bank or credit union sends you a bill they are telling you how much money you owe. That amount is also being sent to the credit reporting agency, which uses it to calculate your credit utilization rate. If your balance is $500 and you owe $500 then your utilization rate is 100% and that's going to look really bad on your credit report. It's going to lower your score by quite a bit.

What you want to do is make more than one payment per month. If your balance at the end of the month is lower than the limit then you're going to have a better utilization rate. The lower the rate you have the better it's going to look on your score, so make sure that you're paying as much as you can for each of your payments. That way, no matter when your credit card company sends in the balance owed, you won't get a big hit on your credit report and you'll be able to keep your score higher, where you want it to be.

www.ingramcontent.com/pod-product-compliance
Lightning Source LLC
Chambersburg PA
CBHW071353280526
45787CB00001B/303